The Chronic Fatigue Syndrome Epidemic Cover-up

Volume Two

The Origins of Totalitarianism in
Science and Medicine

Charles Ortleb

Distributed by Rubicon Media, Salem, Massachusetts

PRINTED IN THE UNITED STATES OF AMERICA

ISBN: 978-0-9983709-2-7

10 9 8 7 6 5 4 3 2 1
First Edition

Contents

The Architects

How Three American Scientists Helped Create
the Nazi Science of Holocaust II

Introduction

If justice and truth prevail in the world, one day what has been called "AIDS" will be renamed "Holocaust II." While gay people were secondary victims of what is referred to as "The Holocaust," or "Holocaust I," they were the main attraction in "Holocaust II." The heterosexist motivation of their stigmatization and persecution in both holocausts were similar even if the manner in which they were harmed was different. I have coined the term "Iatrogenocide" to describe what happened to gay men (and others) during Holocaust II.

I was a witness to the AIDS epidemic from the very beginning. As the publisher and editor-in-chief of *New York Native*, I inadvertently oversaw the reporting of the very first story about the epidemic. After hearing about a strange pneumonia occurring in gay men in New York City, I asked a physician to make inquiries with the public health authorities. In a story headlined "Disease Rumors Largely Unfounded" published in our May 18, 1981 issue, Dr. Lawrence Mass wrote, "Last week there were rumors that an exotic new disease had hit the gay community in New York. Here are the facts. From the New York City Department of Health, Dr. Steve Phillips explained that the rumors are for the most part unfounded. Each year, approximately 12 to 24 cases of infection with a protozoa-like organism, Pneumocystis carinii, are reported in the New York City area. The organism is not exotic; in fact, it's ubiquitous. But most of us have a natural or easily acquired immunity."

Six weeks later it turned out that the rumors were true when the CDC reported on the first cases of what would be called AIDS. It is hard to overstate the shock and terror that gripped the gay community in New York City and eventually around the world. People dreaded waking up each morning as bad news just got worse and worse. Given that my paper seemed to be at the ground zero of the event, I made the conscious decision to devote *New York Native* to covering every detail of the story. For the first two years our coverage was so thorough that some people started referring to my newspaper as "The New York Native Journal of Medicine." Many of our readers and advertisers resented our coverage and wanted us to focus on positive stories. But I felt that we had a responsibility get to the bottom of what was going on.

As the cases mounted and the gay community began to accept the reality of the epidemic, our coverage began to be appreciated and *New York Native* became a trusted source for the latest news about AIDS. In the April 25, 1985 issue of *Rolling Stone*, David Black said that *New York Native* deserved a Pulitzer Prize for our reporting. In his bestselling book, *And the Band Played On*, Randy Shilts wrote, "Because of the extraordinary reporting of the *New York Native*, the city's gay community had been exposed to far more information about AIDS than San Francisco in 1981 and 1982." And in the March 23, 1989 *Rolling Stone*, Katie Leishman wrote, "It is undeniable that many major AIDS stories were Ortleb's months and sometimes years before mainstream journalists took them up." But that love affair with *New York Native* was about to end abruptly.

As I have detailed in my history of *New York Native*, *The Chronic Fatigue Syndrome Epidemic Cover-up*, as the epidemic went on and our reporting became more investigative, I began to notice serious credibility gaps in what the Centers for Disease Control was telling the public about the AIDS epidemic. AIDS increasingly reminded me of the period of egregious government mendacity that occurred during the Vietnam era. As the government began to build a paradigm around the notion that AIDS was caused by a retrovirus ultimately labelled "HIV," I watched as credible critics of the retroviral theory were silenced and vilified. I discuss the heroic voices that spoke out in *The Duesbergians*.

My newspaper became even more controversial when we began reporting on another epidemic called chronic fatigue syndrome. From our extensive reporting, it was hard not to conclude that chronic fatigue syndrome is part of the AIDS epidemic and is linked to AIDS by a virus called HHV-6 which government scientists refused to take seriously.

As AIDS activists increasingly lined up behind the government's HIV/AIDS paradigm and draconian public health agenda, the inconvenient truths my newspaper was reporting about HHV-6 and chronic fatigue syndrome became increasingly unpopular. Nobody wanted to believe that the elite AIDS doctors and scientists might have gotten AIDS totally wrong. Act Up, New York's powerful AIDS activist group, voted to boycott *New York Native* and they did anything they could to put us out of business. Finally, in January 1997, we published our final issue.

In the last twenty years, I have given a great deal of thought to the nature of what happened to my newspaper and to the integrity of AIDS science and medicine. A number of my thoughts on the subject are collected in *Iatrogenocide: Notes for a Political Philosophy of Epidemiology and*

Science. I have also written a play about the politics of the epidemic called *The Black Party*. My thoughts about the racial politics of AIDS can be found in a novella, *The Closing Argument*.

I have come to the conclusion that the similarities between AIDS science and Nazi science are too obvious for people of conscience to ignore. In his groundbreaking book about Nazi treatment of Jews, *"Life Unworthy of Life": Racial Phobia and Mass Murder in Hitler's Germany*, James M. Glass writes, "It was not cultural propagandists who organized the infamous 'special treatment' of the Jews; it was the public health officials, the scientific journals, the physicians, the administrators, and the lawyers, who feared the very presence of the Jews would endanger their families, their bodies, and ultimately their lives. To think of the Jew in such terms is insane from our perspective, but it was held to be sane in the culture caught up in the phobic projection of infection onto the Jews and the scientific authority legitimizing such beliefs." In many ways AIDS, or what I call "Holocaust II," involved what could be called "special epidemiological treatment" of the gays which was created and supported by health officials, scientific journals, physicians, administrators, lawyers, activists, celebrities, and many others. While the manner in which AIDS is understood by public health authorities and the general public is assumed to be sane, a closer look reveals that a genocidal insanity lurks beneath the surface. In the case of AIDS, a fraudulent and phobic epidemiology has been used to scapegoat and biomedically persecute the gay community. And many others.

In this book, I discuss three scientists who I consider to be among the important "architects" of Holocaust II. Each of them played an important role in creating the kind of science which I describe in *Iatrogenocide* as being abnormal, totalitarian, and sociopathic.

Also in *Iatrogenoicde*, I coined the term "homodemiology" to describe the kind of epidemiology that scapegoats gay people for epidemics. I describe the homodemiological politics of the Centers for Disease Control in *The Four Doctors of the Apocalypse*. While the CDC got the ball rolling, I don't think the homodemiological dystopia of Holocaust II would have happened with the contributions of Myron Essex, Anthony Fauci, and Robert Gallo.

Anyone who is reading this book may be tempted to think I am writing about a problem that only affects gay people. That is far from the truth. The frauds of these three scientists have helped conceal an epidemic of a virus called HHV-6 which threatens everyone. Since 2005, at HHV-6 University, I have been covering the biomedical damage that HHV-6 is doing to people all over the world. I have called HHV-6 "The AIDSdromeda Strain" and "The Fifty Shades of AIDS Virus." HHV-6 is a pandemic threatening everyone which has been hidden behind the political mask of HIV/AIDS fraud.

While the first Holocaust may have been focused on Jews, the whole world paid a terrible price for the anti-Semitism that fueled it. In *The Jew as Pariah*, Hannah Arendt wrote, "The comity of European peoples went to pieces when, and because, it allowed its weakest member to be excluded and persecuted." I hope Arendt will forgive me for arguing that the comity and health of the whole world is going to pieces because it is allowing its weakest member (the gay community) to be epidemiologically excluded, scapegoated, and persecuted.

How Harvard's Myron Essex Laid the Groundwork for the Pseudoscience of Holocaust II

FOCMA happened in the decade before the beginning of what could be called "Holocaust II" and the HHV-6 catastrophe, but it was a scientific omen of things to come. One could say that the decline and fall of American biomedical science had a dry run in the FOCMA episode at Harvard. In many ways Harvard was the ground zero for the pseudoscience and retroviral fraud of "Holocaust II."

FOCMA stands for "feline oncornavirus-associated cell-membrane antigen," and it was supposedly discovered in 1977 and named by Myron T. "Max" Essex, a Harvard School of Public Health researcher. According to *Chicago Tribune* reporter John Crewdson, Essex, when he was a post doc, came up with the idea that 'white blood cells from cats infected with the feline leukemia virus also exhibited a unique protein on their surface, "and Essex dubbed that protein 'FOCMA.'" (*Science Fictions* p. 40)

In *Science Fictions*, Crewdson's book on the questionable AIDS research of Robert Gallo, he notes that the importance of Essex's putative discovery was that "If FOCMA were a by-product of the cell's infection with feline leukemia virus, it might represent confirmation of a cellular defense against cancer, at least in cats. . ." (*SF* p. 40) This would have been a major scientific breakthrough, *if* true.

Unfortunately for a junior researcher who decided to devote the early part of his career to the study of FOCMA, it turned out *not* to be what Essex thought it was. The researcher, Wolf Prensky, discovered—to the great detriment of his budding career—that FOCMA "was just a viral protein and not a cellular antigen." (*SF* p.41) According to Crewdson, Prensky, with two other scientists, published a paper "that was a definitive demonstration that the FOCMA protein was encoded by the feline leukemia virus itself, not a cellular by-product of infection." (*SF* p.41) Crewdson notes that "The idea that cat blood cells had some built-in defense against cancer evaporated overnight." (*SF* p.41)

While this matter might seem like an esoteric issue only of concern to the priesthood of science, what happened next was a foreshadowing of the totalitarian culture of abnormal science that would happen throughout the three decades of the scientific shenanigans known as HIV/AIDS. And it would involve some of the same characters. The head of the National Cancer Institute, Vincent DeVita, "selected [Robert] Gallo, despite his co-authorship of a FOCMA article with Essex two years before, to head an investigation of Prensky's claims." (*SF* p.41) This is the kind of little game that would be known throughout "Holocaust II" as "Henhouse, meet Fox."

While the committee came to the conclusion that neither undermined Essex or vindicated him, because, according to Crewdson, *Gallo claimed he didn't understand FOCMA—something he had co-authored a paper about*, a pattern was set of old boys performing due diligence on their own old boy networks. If this was the musical overture for three decades of AIDS science, one could call the melody "sham peer review" and "egregious conflict of interest."

Prensky's career was viciously sidetracked for many years for daring to challenge Essex, and perhaps most importantly, for getting anywhere near what some people eventually considered one of the most dangerous black holes in science: Robert Gallo.

Crewdson, who paradoxically supported the Gallo HIV theory of AIDS despite writing an epic exposé of Gallo that makes Gallo look like the greatest pathological liar in the history of science, doesn't dwell on the FOCMA matter much or with any great outrage, perhaps because Essex's subsequent career would eventually have what Crewdson considered a happy scientific ending due to his peripheral early involvement with HTLV-III, the virus that was officially declared by the government and the AIDS establishment to be the real cause of AIDS in 1984. Crewdson writes that "rather than withdrawing or correcting his FOCMA articles, Essex simply stopped referring to them in his subsequent publications." (*SF* p. 41) He *disappeared* the episode. Crewdson doesn't write a single word about the tremendous damage done to Prensky's career which was the price he paid for telling the truth about one of Essex's discoveries. Prensky's fate foreshadowed the fate of Peter Duesberg, the scientist who would eventually be severely punished for basically saying that HIV was about as much the cause of AIDS as FOCMA was a cellular protection against cancer.

Insofar as Essex just left his "discovery" floating like the undead in the scientific literature without ever retracting it, this little incident of uncorrected science was akin to the broken window theory of crime, in that it may have led to bigger evasions of the truth with far greater implications for mankind. And it also foreshadowed the degree to which both Essex and Gallo would have amazing political and "scientific" power that would allow them to survive and even thrive financially during "Holocaust II." FOCMA was the grain of sand in which one could see the whole universe of HIV/AIDS fraud.

Journalist Barry Werth wrote about FOCMA in an article called "The AIDS Windfall" in *New England Monthly* in June, 1988. He writes that "Dozens of scientists went off in pursuit of FOCMA. But no one could prove that FOCMA existed. Essex abandoned the subject, and he refused to pursue the criticism of those following it up, or to retract it. He simply let FOCMA hang, and other scientists were understandably incensed. 'We'd have figured it out ten years earlier if Essex had only done his homework,' complains one researcher."

Essex was able to move on without ever having to admit he had made a mistake. Werth notes that Essex was able to conveniently change the subject from FOCMA to HTLV: "Essex's work connecting HTLV with AIDS was published in the spring of 1983." The actual so-called AIDS retrovirus, HTLV-III, was a year away from being declared the official cause of AIDS, but Essex had helped pave the way to, depending on your point of view, the Nobel-worthy notion or "Big Mistake" that AIDS was caused by a retrovirus. Werth writes that "the AIDS virus was a retrovirus, just as Essex had said. He's been wrong in all the particulars, but right in general, and being half right secured him the undisputed mantle as the prophet of AIDS." Or as the perpetually witty HIV critic Peter Duesberg might say, the prophet of the most tragic scientific boondoggle in history.

Given Essex's financial and career interest in maintaining the legitimacy of the notion that a retrovirus was the cause of AIDS, it shouldn't surprise anyone that he played an intense enforcement role during the next three decades by helping to elbow out anyone or any that threatened the hegemony of the HIV theory of AIDS. His willingness to play power politics would be dramatically in evidence at the 1992 International AIDS Conference in Amsterdam at which several scientists announced that they had discovered cases of AIDS in which there was *no evidence of HIV*. It didn't take long for the HIV establishment to realize that such cases could turn their retroviral empire into a falling house of cards overnight. In what could be called one of the greatest games of scientific three-card monte, and in the true spirit of abnormal, totalitarian science, the Centers for Disease Control and the powerful HIV establishment effectively swept the paradigm-challenging anomalies under the rug by giving the HIV-negative AIDS cases a new category and a brand new complicated name, idiopathic CD4 T-lymphocytopenia (ICL)."

Because the very embarrassing HIV-negative cases were found *outside* the so-called risk groups, they just couldn't be AIDS. It was a classic instance of circular homodemiological groupthink. *If it wasn't gay, it wasn't AIDS*. Case closed. When researcher Subhir Gupta reported at the 1992 conference that he had found evidence of a retrovirus other than HIV in a sixty-six-year-old woman who had AIDS-like symptoms, but was negative for HIV, Essex stepped right up to the plate. Gupta had published his findings in the *Proceedings of the National Academy of Science*. The findings should have inspired an emergency rethinking of AIDS epidemiology and virology. In *Osler's Web*, Hillary Johnson described the whole incident: "Max Essex, a Harvard AIDS researcher, expressed skepticism bordering on ennui. 'I'm not overwhelmed by it,' he commented after reading the paper. 'I'd place the odds at five to ten percent that this might lead to something.'" (*OW* p.601) (The odds, of course, were nearly 100 percent that Essex would do what he could so that such an outcome was not achieved.) According to Johnson, "Both [David] Ho and Essex raised the specter of laboratory contamination in the matter of Gupta's findings. Microbes such as Gupta described, they said, were notorious laboratory contaminants and could easily have come from an animal cell line." (*OW*. p.601) The AIDS establishment's findings always tended to be scientifically unquestionable (and miraculously contaminant-free) but any findings that challenged the HIV paradigm tended to be contaminants, artifacts, irrelevant correlations. Only the inner circle's labs were pristine and above suspicion.

The very threatened CDC stepped in and quickly reassured the shocked world that there was *not* a new virus causing *another* AIDS epidemic. (This was also at the same time they were—by ignoring it—indirectly assuring the public that there wasn't a contagious immune-system compromising chronic fatigue syndrome epidemic in the general population. In retrospect, and full of the irony that "Holocaust II" is replete with, they were right. It wasn't a new AIDS epidemic, it was part and parcel of the old one, *the one they had gotten the epidemiology and virology wrong on*.) When the CDC's director of AIDS Research, James Curran, told the press that the cases of HIV-negative AIDS like illness were not "AIDS caused by something else," he was just whistling in the dark while HHV-6 spectrum pandemic was having its insidious way with the world and creating a disaster that could not be seen by the abnormal and totalitarian science that was generated by the CDC's homodemiological vision of the epidemic.

From his position on the Mt. Olympus of AIDS, Essex had done his part at that Amsterdam AIDS Conference to help the HIV establishment avoid a crisis of confidence and keep a lid on the horrifying truth about *the real epidemic*. He saved his reputation as the prophet who knew what kind of virus caused AIDS. The coming decades would be a professional dream come true for the man who discovered the nonexistent FOCMA. "Holocaust II" and The Age of Totalitarian, Abnormal and Sociopathic Science could not have existed without Harvard's Myron Essex. He has secured Harvard's place in the history of AIDS fraud.

Anthony Fauci, the Bernie Madoff of Holocaust II

November 2, 1984 was an especially tragic day in the Chronic Fatigue Syndrome/AIDS epidemic. That was the day Anthony Fauci became the Director of the National Institutes of Allergy and Infectious Diseases. (NIAID). (*Good Intentions* p.128) It was the day a thin-skinned, physically ultra-diminutive man with a legendary Napoleonic attitude was positioned by destiny to become the de facto AIDS Czar. In the fog of culpability that constitutes what could be called "Holocaust II" one thing is clear: the buck, on its way to the very top of the government, at least pauses at the megalomaniac desk of Anthony Fauci.

In his book, *Good Intentions*, Bruce Nussbaum writes, "Fauci looked as if he had just stepped out of a limousine. Trim and athletic, Fauci's tailored suits, cuff-linked shirts, and aviator glasses set him far apart from the rest of the scientists and administrators at the NIH." (*GI* p.128) Fauci had risen quickly at NIH. According to Nussbaum, he began work at NIH in 1968 after his residency and "by 1977 he was deputy clinical director of NIAID." (*GI* p.128) Nussbaum describes Fauci as "an aggressive administrator," not a "details man," "a big picture kind of guy." (*GI* p.128) Nussbaum reports that "Fauci saw AIDS as a dreadful disease—and an opportunity for NIAID to grow into a much bigger, more powerful institute. AIDS was his big chance. He wasn't known as a brilliant scientist, and he had little background in managing a big bureaucracy; but Fauci did have ambition and drive to spare. This lackluster scientist was about to find his true vocation—empire building." (*GI* p.128) Unfortunately, the empire his extreme ambition would build was "Holocaust II." If the mantra during Watergate was "follow the money," the mantra for uncovering the crimes of "Holocaust II" (other than "follow the heterosexism") could be "follow the empire building." And one of the morals of the story is that "lackluster" can have extreme consequences.

According to Nussbaum, in order to make his dreams come true, Fauci had to fight "for a bigger piece of the AIDS research pie" which he succeeded at by getting a sizable amount of the funds that Congress appropriated for AIDS research. (*GI* p.129) Fauci also had to fight to get AIDS out of the claws of the National Cancer Institute where the virus that was believed to be the cause of AIDS had been discovered (or, more accurately, stolen). Fauci argued that it was his institute's right to take on the lion's share of the research because, although AIDS did involve cancer (Kaposi's sarcoma), it was, after all, an infectious disease. Fauci got his way and his success is reflected in the evolving financial numbers Nussbaum provides: "A growing budget for AIDS research, like a rising tide, lifted Tony Fauci's profile considerably on the NIH campus. In 1982, NIAID received $297,000 in AIDS funding. In 1986 it received $63 million. In 1987, the sum reached $146 million. By 1990, NIAID's annual AIDS funding was pushing half a billion dollars. Tony Fauci's ship had come in." (*GI* p.132)

Fauci's ship coming in meant the gay community's would be sinking fast. It would fall to Anthony Fauci to be the Enforcer-in-Chief of the "homodemiological" HIV/AIDS and "chronic fatigue syndrome is not AIDS" paradigms of "Holocaust II." No one can argue that he didn't do a spectacular job of paradigm enforcement for three dreadful decades.

Starting in the mid-1980s, an organization called the American Foundation for AIDS Research (amfAR) played a multifaceted role of raising money for HIV research and enlisting celebrities in a glamorous and ultimately shameful HIV propaganda campaign that made the putatively private organization essentially a de facto arm of the government's HIV/AIDS establishment. If one considers the HIV theory of AIDS a Potemkin biomedical village that gays were forced to live in, then amfAR is one of its leading real estate agents. John Lauritsen, in his book, *The AIDS War*, writes that "[amfAR] was founded as an alternative to the AIDS establishment, to provide funding for research that was *not* predicated on the 'AIDS virus' hypothesis. It didn't last long. . . . I am not aware that even a penny has ever been given to a researcher who publicly expressed doubts as to the etiological role of HIV or the benefits of the nucleoside analogues." (*AW* p.437)

In addition to becoming one of the leading private promoters of the government's HIV/AIDS paradigm propaganda, amfAR played a disturbing role in squelching serious scientific criticism of the HIV hypothesis and in helping turn the entire field of AIDS into a world of heterosexist, totalitarian, and abnormal science. Lauritsen describes an historically important amfAR moment in the AIDS disaster in his first book *Poison by Prescription*: "A 'Scientific Forum on the Etiology of AIDS,' sponsored by the American Foundation for AIDS Research (amfAR), was held on 9 April 1988 at the George Washington University in Washington, D.C. In the words of the amfAR 'fact sheet', the forum was convened to critically examine the evidence that human immunodeficiency virus (HIV) or other agents give rise to the disease complex known as AIDS." (*PBP* p.143)

According to Lauritsen, it was supposedly an opportunity for Peter Duesberg, the University of California at Berkeley retrovirologist who first challenged the HIV theory of AIDS "to confront members of the 'AIDS Establishment' over their hypothesis." (*PBP* p.143) He reports, however, that "Despite these praiseworthy intentions, the forum appears to have had a hidden agenda; to discredit Duesberg." (*PBP* p.143) Lauritsen characterized the forum as a "Kangaroo Court." The forum would make a great scene in a play about the nasty, zany world of AIDS and HIV pseudoscience. It was anything but an honest, open collegial discussion about the nature of AIDS. Scientific philosopher Thomas Kuhn would roll over in his grave if anyone called it genuinely scientific. By Kuhn's standards, some of the leading voices at the forum may have even demonstrated that they should not even have been considered real scientists. Politicians, yes, scientists not so much. Even the HIV theory's ardent acolyte, Michael Specter, the reporter from *The Washington Post* (and future *New Yorker* writer) who was among the 17 journalists at the Forum, saw through the charade, noting that the meeting "was billed as a scientific forum on the cause of AIDS but was really an attempt to put Duesberg's theories to rest." (*PBP* p.144) It was more like they wanted to put Duesberg himself permanently to rest.

The meeting had the tone and style that was endemic to HIV/AIDS research and characteristic of abnormal and totalitarian science. Lauritsen reported, "While no blows were struck, some of the HIV protagonists fell below the standards of civility that are expected in scholarly debate. At all times Duesberg retained good manners and a sense of humor, in the face of invective, insults, and clowning from his opponents." (*PBP* p.144)

One of the signs that AIDS in general was being conducted in the opposite world of what could be called abnormal, totalitarian science was the uncanny willingness of the scientists to abandon the traditional rules of evidence known as Koch's postulates. Instead, AIDS researchers, including the ones at the amfAR forum, were willing to "revise Koch's in a more permissive direction: it would no longer be necessary to find the microbe in all cases of the disease. Mere correlations between microbial *antibodies* and the progression of the disease would be sufficient. HIV could be proved 'epidemiologically' to be the cause of AIDS." (*PBP* p.145) Given the unrecognized sexual politics of the science that was operative among this crowd, they were basically saying, without realizing it, that causation could be established "*homodemiologically*." The presumptions of heterosexist and political epidemiology would trump the traditional rules of evidence. And those rules could basically be summed up as "Heads I win and tails you lose." "You" basically being gays and eventually blacks.

Lauritsen caught the powerful HIV advocates in the act of doublespeak that is common to abnormal, totalitarian science: "Actually, the HIV advocates talked out of both sides of their mouths with regard to Koch's postulates. On the one hand, they disparaged them as in need of 'modification' (read abandonment); on the other hand, they were doing their best to come up with data that would satisfy at least the first postulate." (*PBP* p.145)

Duesberg's opponents at the forum included a living, breathing example of scientific conflict of interest, William Haseltine, a scientist who was in the process of making a lot of money from HIV testing, and Anthony Fauci, the empire-building Director of NIAID.

At the amfAR Forum, Fauci and others played a curious unfair game with Duesberg. Hypocritically they accused Duesberg of citing research that was out of date even though it was basically *the same research quoted at that time* by the AIDS establishment. On the other hand, when Duesberg would ask Fauci and others for actual references to support *their* statements at the amfAR forum, he was "rudely rebuffed," and according to Lauritsen, they tried to shore up their viewpoint about HIV with unpublished data, or "their own private facts." (*PBP* p.147) "Private facts" not on the public record are another sure sign that AIDS was a manifestation of the opposite world of abnormal, totalitarian and sociopathic science. Unfortunately, their private facts about AIDS were also connected to each other by a private scientific logic.

The 800-pound gorilla at the amfAR forum was the fact that evidence of HIV *could not be found in all AIDS patients*, which should have been strong—damning even—evidence that HIV couldn't possibly be the cause of AIDS, that is, if Kuhnian normal science was being practiced. As scientist Marcel Beluda pointed out at the meeting, "sometimes even a single exception is sufficient to disprove a theory. . . . This is the crux of the matter. The virus cannot be found in all cases of AIDS." (*PBP* p.151) One could say that still believing that HIV is the cause of AIDS in the face of evidence that it could not be found in all patients is Exhibit A that delusion and denial were running the show.

Fauci's answer belongs in a beginner's textbook on the card tricks of abnormal science: "Fauci responded to Beluda by saying that a good lab was able to isolate the virus in 90-100% of the cases, that there was 'no question about it.' Fauci did not provide a reference to published data, nor did he indicate what the 'good labs' were, or how exactly they differed from the not-so-good labs." (*PBP* p.151) References belong to the abandoned Kuhnian world of normal science.

Duesberg made a number of arguments, based on his years as one of the celebrated deans of retroviral research, about why HIV could not possibly be the cause of AIDS.

Lauritsen wrote that Fauci's presentation "while aspiring to be a point-by-point rebuttal to Duesberg, consisted mainly of disconnected assertions, delivered in a tone of petulant indignation. Epidemiological studies conducted in San Francisco and unpublished laboratory reports seemed to be the basis of most of his statements. So far as I could tell, he understood none of Duesberg's arguments . . . ." (*PBP* p.155)

The role of the AIDS politics of epidemiology in AIDS research showed itself dramatically at the forum. According to Lauritsen, "In the question period, Beluda asked if the evidence were sufficient that HIV is necessary for the development of AIDS, Fauci replied that he hoped the epidemiologists would answer that question." (*PBP* p.157) (Given the political and heterosexist nature of AIDS epidemiology, one could guess how *that* was going to turn out.)

The most shocking and downright hilarious episode at the forum occurred when Harvard Medical School's William Haseltine spoke. Lauritsen reported that "His presentation was devoted largely to personal attacks on Duesberg." (*PBP* p.157) Ironically, *he* accused Duesberg of resorting to personal attacks. In another telltale moment of abnormal and totalitarian science, Lauritsen caught Haseltine trying to explain away the anomalies about the evidence of AIDS in men and women in America: "He attacked Duesberg's 'paradox,' that the AIDS virus seemed to be able to discriminate between boys and girls, by saying that this was not true outside the U.S.—in Africa, about equal numbers of men and women develop AIDS. (He seemed oblivious to the paradox that a microbe should be able to discriminate in one country, but not in another.)" (*PBP* p.158) In a memorable moment that perfectly captured the essence of the past and future of AIDS research, Haseltine showed the audience a slide of a graph that was meant to absolutely demolish Duesberg's argument. The slide was supposed to show a correlation between the rise in HIV titers with the decline of T cells in the progression of AIDS. There was just one small problem: Duesberg quickly noticed that *there were no units on the vertical axis of the slide.* Haseltine was angry and flustered by the charge and had to ask Dr. Robert Redfield, an AIDS researcher from the military, how the slide was prepared. At the forum Redfield said, "different measurements were used," but later that night at a post-forum party, according to Lauritsen's report, Redfield told Duesberg and other people at the gathering that "the graph had been prepared to illustrate a theoretical possibility. It had no units on it for the simple reason that *it was not based on any data at all.* In other words, the slide was a fake." (*PBP* p.161) That's the kind of ideology-based data that was used to back up the HIV theory of AIDS which changed the course of millions of lives and fostered the HHV-6 catastrophe.

In terms of the habitual use of political epidemiology (or "homo-demiology") rather than real science to deal with AIDS during "Holocaust II," the most disturbing talk was given by Warren Winkelstein, Professor of Biomedical Environmental Health Sciences at U.C. Berkeley. Essentially, he too suggested that AIDS would require *a new kind of science.* According to Lauritsen, "the point of Winkelstein's presentation is that Koch's postulates should be superseded by new standards for establishing the causal relationship between microbes and disease, and that these standards should be based upon 'epidemiology' or, as it were, correlations of various kinds." (*PBP* p.162) If this crowd had superseded traditional science any more than they did, we all would probably be dead. (But wait. There is still time.)

Most of the scientific world was not aware of the degree to which this zany cast of characters was improvising a questionable newfangled science as they went along. And it was being done in a Fauci-style of "petulant indignation," to reprise Lauritsen's very apt phrase. That it was all dependent on a loosey-goosey, all too subjective political "discipline" like epidemiology should have disturbed Lauritsen's sixteen journalistic colleagues who were at the amfAR affair. But there was already a tragically cozy relationship between the media and the abnormal, totalitarian and sociopathic scientists of "Holocaust II." For three decades as the HIV/AIDS paradigm held sway, most of the reporters who covered AIDS were a self-satisfied, inattentive, group-thinking, intellectually slothful bunch who wouldn't know independent, journalistic due diligence if it bit them. A corrupt scientific community could totally depend on them.

Lauritsen's eyewitness record of the forum (originally published in *New York Native*) was an important contribution to the history of the flakey beginnings of the science and totalitarian politics of AIDS. His diligent and critical reporting is proof that *not every journalist* was hoodwinked by these charlatans. He didn't buy into this new improvised epidemiological science that the AIDS establishment was dumping on the public: "I do not accept the proposition that Koch's postulates should be abandoned in favor of epidemiological correlations. This would be a step backward, a step away from scientific rigor, a step towards impressionism and confusion." (*PBP* p.162) Lauritsen didn't acknowledge it, but it was also a big heterosexist (and ultimately racist) step backwards.

Like many others, Lauritsen came face to face with totalitarian, abnormal, and sociopathic science. Unfortunately, even though he was openly gay himself, he didn't grasp the manner in which the infernal game was being played—or what the game was actually concealing. He didn't fully perceive the homodemiological underpinnings of what was happening before his very eyes. But he definitely grasped the fact that the science of the budding AIDS Establishment was utterly bogus. He concluded his report by writing, "I am more convinced than ever that HIV is not the cause of AIDS. If the HIV advocates were sure of their hypothesis, they would want to enlighten Duesberg and the rest of us; they would want to publish their arguments in a proper scientific journal complete with references. They would not need to resort to stonewalling, deception, and personal abuse." (*PBP* p.168) Science had been supplanted by totalitarian petulance.

The 1988 amfAR Forum was another one of the tragic "What if?" moments in the dark history of AIDS. What if the reporters had looked closer at Haseltine's fake slide and realized that it was the tip of the iceberg, a little like the scientific version of the Watergate break-in that would have led them to a much bigger crime if they only followed the lies? What if they had reported that AIDS science, as practiced by Anthony Fauci, was simply out-to-lunch? What if they had been independent enough to notice that epidemiology was overplaying its arrogant, biased hand and that, in reality, it is actually a soft, subjective enterprise vulnerable to political manipulation? Why was it beyond the pale to wonder if this defensive and cranky gathering was actually the expression of some rather unsavory feelings and hostilities directed at the so-called beneficiaries of this new kind of "science," namely the gay community? Maybe someone should have asked if there was something funky about a group of hostile, arrogant, white heterosexual mostly-male scientists performing their jerry-built kind of seat-of-the-pants epidemiological science on gays. Wasn't that a formula for all kinds of prurient, heterosexist pseudoscientific mischief if ever there was one? In terms of majorities doing their science on minorities, hadn't anyone ever heard of Nazi science or the Tuskegee Syphilis Experiment? God only knows what personal sexual issues were being acted out by this elite motley crew under the cover of what has turned out to be highfalutin retroviral claptrap. Why didn't anyone other than Lauritsen notice the peculiar, unscientific defensiveness of the whole affair, i.e. that the ladies had protested too much? And most importantly for the main event, why was HHV-6, which had been discovered in AIDS patients two years before that curious amfAR forum, not put on the table for discussion?

Fauci believed in the kind of transparency and communications with the public that are typical of abnormal science. He laid out the draconian media policy that he would maintain for the nearly thirty years he ran the totalitarian HIV/AIDS empire in a brief piece he wrote for the AAAS Observer on September 1, 1989.

Fauci wrote, "When I first got involved in AIDS research, I was reluctant to deal with the press. I thought it was not dignified. But there was a lot of distortion by those who were speaking to the press so I changed my mind." The "distortion" was, of course, coming from those who didn't agree with the very dignified Fauci about the etiology of AIDS. Fauci had his own idea of what the media's responsibility is. He notes that his interpretation of what the media is supposed to do "doesn't even jibe with what competent journalists think." He asserts that the big dilemma for journalists is between what is "important" and what is "newsworthy" and he notes that they sometimes "are not the same." He whines about the fact that journalists are more interested in the latest story of a cure than the "magnificent science" involving the regulatory genes of HIV.

Fauci describes what he thinks is the hierarchy of media. It ranges from *The New York Times* and *The Washington Post* all the way down to publications that "care only about sales or have axes to grind." (He had yet to face the unwashed barbarians of the blogs and the commenters of the online forums.) One can safely assume that the publications with axes to grind were the ones who didn't agree with the axe that the petulant Fauci himself was grinding. It is amusing that Fauci pontificated in 1989 that "the media are no place for amateurs, particularly when talking about a public health problem of the magnitude of AIDS." Especially when one considers the magnitude of the HHV-6 public health problem that this very self-reverential scientist (that Bruce Nussbaum described as "lackluster") himself helped create for the whole human race. While Fauci would make one think that the real problem in AIDS journalism was the clownish journalist who can't spell "retrovirus" or one who didn't listen carefully after asking questions, his real quarry in this peevish little piece is something far more serious. Fauci's real problem was journalists who not only *could* spell "retrovirus" but could also actually hear what he was saying *all too well*. The kind of journalists who also knew things about retroviruses and listened to what he was saying so closely and critically that they could make life unpleasant for Fauci and his powerful AIDS cronies by asking inconvenient questions.

Fauci's nose should have grown several feet when he wrote, "We know that reporters must consult more than a single source and make room for dissenting opinions." What was yet to come in the AAAS piece made that one of the biggest fibs in the history of American science. Under the pretense of giving us a little lesson in the relationship between science and the media and warning that people too often believe what they read in the papers, Fauci reveals his real agenda: "One striking example is Peter Duesberg's theory that HIV is not the cause of AIDS. I laughed at that for a while, but it led to a lot of public concern that HIV was a hoax. The theory had a great deal of credibility just on the basis of news coverage." This was Fauci being intellectually dishonest on a couple of counts. Duesberg never said it was a *hoax*. He said it was a *mistake*. A hoax is a whole other ball of wax, and it is an example of using language politically to deliberately misrepresent the opposition. Duesberg wasn't saying something similar to those who say that the landing on the moon was just staged with props and a camera. He was a Nobel-caliber expert on retroviruses pointing out the deficiencies of the HIV theory of AIDS using basic logic and analyzing the available evidence. And blaming the media for the credibility given to Duesberg's ideas ignored all the scientists, (eventually including two Nobel Prize winners), who publicly supported Duesberg's skepticism. Fauci was Trumpian in that he was essentially accusing those who spotted his fake science as being purveyors of fake news.

Fauci then introduces us to the smarter member of his family, his sister: "My barometer of what the general public is thinking is my sister Denise. My sister Denise is an intelligent woman who reads avidly, listens to the radio, and watches television, but she is not a scientist. When she calls me and questions my integrity as a scientist, there really is a problem. Denise has called me at least ten times about Peter Duesberg. She says,

'Anthony'—she is the only one who calls me Anthony, 'are you sure he's wrong?' That's the power of putting someone on television or in the press, although there is virtually nothing in his argument that makes any scientific sense." This captures how touchy Fauci was. No one was questioning his "integrity as a scientist." His sister was simply asking him if it was *possible* that he was wrong, and the answer that would have shown some scientific integrity would have been, "Yes, my dear Denise, it is always possible that I'm wrong, although I think the evidence suggests I'm right." The fact that Fauci took this *soooooo* personally speaks volumes about the petulant chip-on-the-shoulder attitude problems of those in charge of AIDS. Fauci put it all on the line. Questioning his so-called science was a threat to his very being. It shouldn't surprise anyone that he was willing to viciously fight for so long during "Holocaust II" to keep everyone from seeing what a house of cards he had helped build. The funny thing is that in a number of ways this scientific masterpiece suggests he *did* have serious problems in the integrity department. (Between the lines of the piece Freudian historians may one day even find the glimmer of a guilty conscience.)

Fauci, like most of the crowd that gave us "Holocaust II," knew only too well what normal, nontotalitarian science is supposed to look like: "People are especially confused when they see divergent viewpoints about the same thing. They do not understand that the beauty of science is that it is self-corroborating and self-correcting, that it is important for scientists to be wrong." (If that's really the case, Fauci *was* indeed doing something incredibly important with HIV.) It was actually Fauci who didn't understand that the whole process of self-corroboration and self-correction was being short-circuited by the totalitarian hijinks of the touchy HIV/AIDS establishment that was growing more dominant by the day. The very tone of Fauci's piece, its extraordinary imperiousness and presumptuousness about the stupidity of the public, points to the fundamental problem for a society in which arrogant and dishonest elite scientific communities have more and more power. Fauci would not only be the judge and jury of what was true in science, but he also wanted to decide *who* deserved to write about it and *what* they should write. He clearly left no room for the possibility that the really good journalists would be the kind that questioned what *he* had to say.

Fauci also made it pretty clear in the piece that, try as they might, AIDS critics and dissidents would get absolutely nowhere because he was permanently stacking the deck against them: "The lack of clear-cut black-or-white answers plagues the biomedical sciences compared with the physical sciences. Stanley Pons and Martin Fleishmann said they had achieved nuclear fusion at room temperature. Other scientists tried, but they could not reproduce it. Bingo it's over. But because we cannot ethically do clinical trials to establish that he is wrong, I am probably going to be answering Peter Duesberg for the rest of my life." Someone near him should have tried to convince Fauci that it wasn't all about *him*. One also loves the presumption that he was going to control the official etiology of AIDS *for the rest of his life*. Unfortunately, *he almost has*. Beyond the breathtaking megalomania of the statement is the stupidity that the only way to show HIV wasn't the cause of AIDS was to do clinical trials with patients. All it would have taken would have been a few patients with AIDS *who had no evidence of HIV*. The only people that would be hurt by the implications of that finding would be the dishonest and incompetent scientists, like Fauci, whose undeserved reputations and incomes had depended upon the HIV theory. Those HIV-negative patients would be forthcoming—in spades. In fact those patients were basically the very immune-compromised chronic fatigue syndrome patients a doctor named Richard DuBois had seen in his Atlanta practice *before* the socio-epidemiological construction of the heterosexist and racist HIV/AIDS paradigm.

Hillary Johnson reported on the DuBois Atlanta cases in *Osler's Web: Inside the Labyrinth of Chronic Fatigue Syndrome Epidemic*, her epic work of journalism detailing the CDC's failure to acknowledge the true nature of the chronic fatigue syndrome epidemic. It is now all too painfully obvious that the DuBois cases—with the telltale signs of hypergamma-globulinemia, t-cell perturbations and persistent reactivated EBV and CMV infections—were the beginning of the real AIDS/CFS/HHV-6 disaster. According to Johnson, in 1980 Richard DuBois "saw a thirteen-year old girl who suffered from a seemingly endless case of mono. As the months passed, he identified several more cases of the curious syndrome in his practice." (*OW* p.7) He wasn't alone. Johnson reported that he was in touch with other clinicians who had seen similar cases and he and his colleagues eventually had a research article published about it in the *Southern Medical Journal* in 1984, the same year the big consequential government mistake of certifying HIV as the official AIDS virus occurred. According to Johnson, "they [DuBois and his colleagues] had believed that they were describing a new syndrome, one that would have increasing importance and was worthy of national attention." (*OW* p.7) The DuBois patients morphed into the millions of chronic fatigue syndrome and HHV-6 patients that Fauci and his organization (which was supposed to handle infectious diseases) were willfully ignoring while building their Potemkin HIV/AIDS empire.

At the end of Fauci's little *AAAS* piece comes the shot across the media's bow from the tiny AIDS czar: "Scientists need to get more sophisticated about expressing themselves. But the media have to do their homework. They have got to learn the issues and the background. And they should realize that their accuracy is noted by the scientific community. Journalists who make too many mistakes, who are sloppy, are going to find that their access to scientists may diminish." In other words, the scientists that journalists reported on were going to be the high-handed and underhanded final arbiters of what the public knows about science. They could decide to cut off journalists *they* defined as making mistakes and being sloppy, and one would assume that one of those sloppy mistakes would probably entail giving coverage to scientists like Peter Duesberg, who raised serious questions about what was being called good science by Fauci and the rest of the HIV/AIDS establishment. Fauci was basically saying that he and his cronies would only be accountable to themselves which is the hermetically-sealed, closed-community essence of what should be called totalitarian, abnormal, and ultimately sociopathic science.

If anyone ever makes a serious film about "Holocaust II" it will have to include the shocking revelation (already referred to above) that came to light during the Eighth International Conference on AIDS in Amsterdam during July of 1992. Its historic importance rivals that of the Wannsee conference during World War II or the Gulf of Tonkin incident. It *was the moment of no turning back*, the moment a fateful line was crossed, a life of virtual pseudoscientific crime against humanity was virtually signed onto and those responsible for "Holocaust II" lost all forms of plausible deniability. AIDS almost overnight became AIDSgate and a very unique Nazi-like biomedical and epidemiological assault against humanity. And, ultimately, the man who stood at the center of the developments that came out of Amsterdam was Anthony Fauci. Before Amsterdam one might be able to say that Fauci wasn't exactly the Bernie Madoff of the biomedical Ponzi Scheme that maintained AIDS, chronic fatigue syndrome and the HHV-6 spectrum catastrophe. *But not after Amsterdam.*

Hillary Johnson provided a detailed account of what happened at that Amsterdam conference in her book. She recounts how the conference was electrified by news from a small press conference that was held in California at which a scientist named "Subhir Gupta, a University of California immunologist, reported he had isolated particles of a previously unknown retrovirus from an HIV-negative, ailing sixty-six-year-old woman, her symptomless daughter and six other patients." (*OW* p.600) According to Johnson, "Investigators and the lay press gathered in Holland were riveted by Gupta's announcement that the older woman suffered from an 'AIDS-like' condition wherein a component of her immune system, a subset of T-cells called CD4 cells, were severely depleted. In addition, she had suffered a bout of *Pneumocystis carinii* pneumonia, a so-called opportunistic infection that afflicted many AIDS patients whose CD4 cells were depleted." (*OW* p.600)

That announcement was soon outdone by a flurry of shocking revelations from additional scientists at the Amsterdam conference who had "findings of retrovirus particles in HIV-negative patients with AIDS-like symptoms." (*OW* p.601) A near panic was almost set off internationally by the possibility that there was a second previously unrecognized AIDS epidemic on the horizon that was caused by a non-HIV agent. (*OW* p.601)

According to Johnson, it turned out that the Centers for Disease Control *was already aware* of such HIV-negative cases of an AIDS-like illness. (*OW* p.601) Johnson reported that months before Gupta's press conference two CDC scientists had reported on "six cases of non-HIV positive AIDS." (*OW* p.601) Their conclusion was that "HIV may not be the only infectious cause of immune deficiency." (*OW* p.601) Two AIDS viruses? A gay one and a straight one? OMG!

The HIV-negative cases of AIDS-like illness set off an explosion in the press, most notably from Lawrence Altman, the reporter who guided *The New York Times* dreadful, sycophantic reporting on AIDS throughout "Holocaust II." In the *Times* Altman wrote that the CDC's embarrassment was "huge because the agency had lost control over the dissemination of new information in the field of AIDS." (*OW* p.602) (That anyone at the *Times* could stress the importance of a government agency *controlling information* with a straight face is pretty amazing and revealing.)

According to Johnson, the CFS research community was especially fascinated by the fact that the Gupta HIV-negative AIDS-like cases were chronic fatigue syndrome sufferers. (*OW* p.604) And for anyone following the bizarre scientific politics of AIDS, it was interesting that Gupta's colleague, the man who supposedly isolated the new retrovirus was none other than Zaki Salahuddin, the scientist who had worked for Robert Gallo and had faced criminal charges for creating a company that garnered illegal self-dealt income from his position at the National Cancer Institute. Johnson reported that when Salahuddin was asked whether HIV-negative

AIDS might be chronic fatigue syndrome, he said, "It's a fair statement. But I'm not a prophet. Time and money [are] required for this." (*OW* p.604) Johnson also reported, "Salahuddin confirmed that he and Gupta, who had a cohort of CFS patients in his clinical practice and who had presented papers on the immunology of CFS at medical conferences on the disease, had discussed the possibility that CFS and non-HIV positive AIDS were the same disease." (*OW* p.604) Also, according to Johnson, the non-HIV positive AIDS cases caught the attention of Paul Cheney, one of the two pioneering Lake Tahoe chronic fatigue syndrome researchers. Johnson wrote, "For years he had observed that some CFS patients met the government's defining criteria for AIDS on every count except infection with human immunodeficiency virus." (*OW* p.604) He also told Johnson that "It was hardly unheard of . . . to diagnose the kinds of opportunistic infections that torment AIDS victims—maladies like thrush, candida and pneumonia—in CFS." (*OW* p.604) In the world of normal science this would have been called "the smoking gun."

The AIDS conference in 1992 should have been one of those great moments in normal science as described by Thomas Kuhn. It could have been a moment when disturbing "anomalies" should have attracted the "attention of a scientific community." (*The Structure of Scientific Revolutions* p.ix) But this would not be a moment for AIDS research that "the profession can no longer evade anomalies that subvert the existing tradition of scientific practice" which would "begin the extraordinary investigations that lead the profession at last to a new set of commitments, a new basis for the practice of science." (*SSR* p.6) This would *not* be one of those eureka moments in science characterized by "the community's rejection of one time-honored scientific theory in favor of another incompatible with it." (*SSR* p.6) There would be no "transformation of the world within which science was done." (*SSR* p.6) There would be no "change in the rules governing the prior practice." (*SSR* p.7) As a result of what happened in Amsterdam, scientists would *not* alter their "conception of entities with which [they] had long been familiar." (*SSR* p.7) Amsterdam would *not* cause the AIDS researchers' worlds to be "qualitatively transformed as well as quantitatively enriched by fundamental novelties of either fact or theory." (*SSR* p.7) After the revelations of HIV-negative AIDS cases, the researchers would still *not* give up their "shared paradigm." (*SSR* p.11) No new AIDS (or chronic fatigue syndrome = AIDS) paradigm was allowed to reveal itself in Amsterdam and subsequently be fairly examined and debated. The HIV-negative cases of AIDS would *not* be recognized as an important scientific surprise that would lead scientists "to see nature in a different way." (*SSR* p.53) The scientific world of AIDS researchers did not change "in an instant" (*SSR* p.56) the way it might have if AIDS research was taking place in the world of normal science. (And consequently, immune-system-destroying HHV-6 would remain locked in the basement of "science.")

Tragically, the HIV-negative AIDS cases were not a wake-up call for the scientists that "something had gone wrong" and hence the anomalous cases were not "a prelude to discovery." (*SSR* p.57) Even though the HIV-negative AIDS cases "violated deeply entrenched expectations," (*SSR* p.59) they were not allowed to change *anything* about the AIDS paradigm. In Kuhn's world of normal science, the "traditional pursuit prepares the way for its own change." (*SSR* p.65) Amsterdam showed that AIDS research was being conducted in normal science's cockamamie opposite world, one that should be called "abnormal, totalitarian and sociopathic science." Even if the HIV-negative AIDS cases could have ultimately led to a new paradigm that was "able to account for wider range of natural phenomena," (*SSR* p.66) they were dead on arrival. No "novel theory" about AIDS which was a "direct response to crisis" (*SSR* p.75) was allowed to emerge because the abnormal, totalitarian, and sociopathic science of AIDS was *politically invulnerable* to crisis. At that historic conference there was never any chance that the HIV/AIDS theory would be "declared invalid" even though a new "CFS is a form of AIDS" paradigm was staring out at the conference from the new anomalous data and was a perfectly credible "alternate candidate." (*SSR* p.77) Kuhn wrote that the decision to reject one paradigm is always simultaneously the decision to accept another, and the judgment leading to that decision involves the comparison of both paradigms with nature and with each other." (*SSR* p.77) The HIV-negative AIDS cases were *not allowed* to catalyze that kind of fertile intellectual process in Amsterdam. Kuhn would probably argue that absent a new paradigm to examine and accept in Amsterdam, there was no exit from the HIV/AIDS paradigm because "To reject one paradigm without simultaneously substituting another is to reject science itself." (*SSR* p.79) In a way, much of what happened at the AIDS conference was based on appeals to something quite characteristic of the AIDS establishment and abnormal science: *authority*. The petulant HIV/AIDS authorities basically said, "Nothing here, folks. Please move along." And unfortunately, the scientific community and the media (with a few notable exceptions) did exactly that. Kuhnian *anomaly* didn't turn into Kuhnian *crisis* and that in turn did not explode into Kuhnian *scientific revolution* as it should have. The HIV-negative cases in Amsterdam should have led to a period of what Kuhn called "extraordinary science" (*SSR* p.82) in which "the rules of normal science become increasingly blurred." (*SSR* p.83) (Although one could argue that the rules of AIDS research already actually were a shocking chocolate mess.) Amsterdam would not be the transformative moment when "formerly standard solutions of solved problems are called into question." (*SSR* p.83) The conference should have been a fruitful time when scientists were "terribly confused." (*SSR* p.84) If things had gone the way they should have at that conference, the assembled AIDS researchers would have ultimately changed their view of "the field, its methods, and its goals." (*SSR* p.85) HHV-6 might have been allowed to reveal itself in all its pathological glory. And the scientists who had given us the HIV paradigm would have been revealed in all their vainglory.

Had the science of Amsterdam been *normal*, both AIDS research and chronic fatigue syndrome research might have morphed into one unified discipline. The dismantling of the "chronic fatigue syndrome isn't AIDS" paradigm should have begun in earnest. HHV-6 (and its spectrum or family) might have emerged quickly as the unifying viral agent(s) of those two epidemics which should have always been considered one in the first place. And those two epidemics were just the tip of the HHV-6 iceberg. What happened in Amsterdam was a virtual nosological and epidemiological crime. It was the deliberate attempt to use *sheer political force* to make a legitimate scientific crisis disappear. As a result, scientists would not turn to what Kuhn describes as a "philosophical analysis as a device for unlocking the riddles of their field." (*SSR* p.88) "Philosophical analysis" was Greek to this confederacy of dunces. The crisis was not allowed to play itself out and would not loosen what Kuhn calls the "stereotypes" and provide "the incremental data necessary for a fundamental paradigm shift." (*SSR* p.89) There would be no Kuhnian "transition from normal to extraordinary research." (*SSR* p.91) It should have been painfully clear in Amsterdam "that an existing paradigm [had] ceased to function adequately in the exploration of an aspect of nature to which that paradigm itself had previously led the way." (*SSR* p.92)

A potentially life-saving scientific revolution in AIDS and CFS research was politically nipped in the bud in Amsterdam and in the months that followed. No "new theory" was allowed to surface that would "permit predictions that are different from those derived from its predecessor" (*SSR* p.97) Kuhn asserted that "the price of significant scientific advance is a commitment that runs the risk of being wrong."(*SSR* p.101) Those in control of the abnormal science of AIDS had no interest in engaging in *any* kind of science that would prove *them* wrong. "Wrong" was not in their cultish vocabulary. They had bet their white heterosexual male professional reputations and the credibility of American science on their ridiculous and dangerous HIV/AIDS and "chronic fatigue syndrome is not AIDS" paradigms. Fake dividends of their scientific Ponzi Scheme would be paid out for decades.

What happened in Amsterdam was the opening and almost simultaneously closing of a Pandora's Box of incredibly important scientific questions and implications. The person most responsible for keeping that box closed then and for the next two decades was the de facto AIDS Czar, the tantrum-prone Anthony Fauci. This may have been the last chance for Fauci and the HIV/AIDS establishment to turn back from the precipice of the HHV-6 spectrum catastrophe. But even his sister Denise could not save him from securing this dark place in history.

According to Hillary Johnson, "On August 15, federal scientists convened a meeting in Atlanta to discuss the emerging health threat of non-HIV positive AIDS. In the three weeks since Sudhir Gupta's paper on his isolation of a new intracisternal retrovirus in a handful of cases, the number of reported cases had risen from approximately thirty to fifty. Nobel prize winners, members of the National Academy of Sciences, CDC's AIDS administrators, and Anthony Fauci, head of the National Institute of Allergy and Infectious Diseases, formed a panel to query scientists Gupta, David Ho of the Aaron Diamond AIDS Center in New York and Jeffrey Laurence, a Cornell Medical College cancer and AIDS specialist and associate professor of medicine, each of whom had been studying cases of the syndrome and discovered evidence of retroviral infection in patients." (*OW* p.606) It didn't matter how many brilliant scientists from different institutions were queried at the meeting, because their mindsets about HIV were all the same. It was like a mini-Woodstock of groupthink. There was no turning back from the HIV/AIDS and "chronic fatigue syndrome *is not* AIDS" paradigm. The carved-in-stone paradigm was eight years old at that point and the nation's heterosexist and racist AIDS propaganda and public health policies had been built on its assumptions. The gay and black communities had been herded into it like cattle into a train. It was another moment in abnormal science in which the privileged and paranoid foxes had formed a panel to investigate the henhouse.

The manner in which Fauci and his colleagues basically covered up the shocking anomalies of HIV-negative AIDS was relatively simple and Orwellian: as previously noted, they disingenuously gave the HIV-negative cases an obfuscational new name (Idiopathic CD4 T lymphocytopenia or ICL) and they insisted by fiat that they were not really AIDS cases. The

HIV/AIDS elite insisted that because there was no unifying geographic or chronological "risk factor" (OW P.603) to be found in these ordinary Americans and they shared no official AIDS risk factors, there was no HIV-negative AIDS or AIDS-like epidemic covertly occurring in the general population. Fauci's concerned sister Denise would not have to lose sleep at night.

Because the "chronic fatigue syndrome *is not* AIDS" paradigm was not challenged by what happened at the Amsterdam Conference in 1992, for at least another two more decades, the chronic fatigue syndrome patients were locked into their pathetic heterosexist wild goose chase to find a cause while constantly avoiding the obvious links between their medical issues and AIDS. They had Tony Fauci's blessing for that fool's errand. His basic attitude toward CFS was that people shouldn't be ashamed of being told that their problem was psychiatric, (*OW* p.334) which was how the disease was deceptively framed by the government for nearly three decades. And of course, they were just the canaries in the HHV-6 mine. Everyone suffering from multi-systemic problems of the HHV-6 spectrum (like multiple sclerosis, fibromyalgia, autism, and even Morgellons) would ultimately pay a heavy price for the intellectual dishonesty and legerdemain of the 1992 AIDS conference.

Fauci and his colleagues told the public that the HIV-negative cases of AIDS-like illness were rare, but of course it all depended on disease definitions and *who* was doing the defining and counting. Fauci disingenuously sent out a call that summer asking that all HIV-negative cases be reported immediately *to him*. An editorial in *New York Native* heeded his call: "Last week Anthony Fauci of the National Institute of Allergy and Infectious Diseases asked that all cases of HIV-negative AIDS be reported to him. We reported thirteen million American cases. That's the estimate of the number of cases of chronic fatigue and immune dysfunction, a condition that research (if anyone bothers to read it) suggests is essentially HIV-negative AIDS." (*OW* p.605)

The editorial had no impact on Anthony Fauci and it would not be the only time he would ignore the *New York Native* during "Holocaust II."

One could ultimately say that Denise Fauci's petulant brother himself represented one of the most significant scientific paradigm shifts, one that moved the whole world from normal to abnormal, totalitarian, and sociopathic science. During the Fauci years, The Age of Scientific Racketeering began in earnest. Bernie Madoff has a twin in science whose Ponzi Scheme is a gift that keeps on giving.

The Pulitzer Prize Winner and
Robert Gallo's Little Lab of Horrors

What the world didn't know, of course, is how much Gallo had done to create the image of an obsessed [*Chicago Tribune* reporter—and chronicler of Robert Gallo's misdeeds—John] Crewdson. Only Crewdson, who recorded the defamation of his character with the same diligence and care that he recorded everything else, knew. He knew it from having to answer when his sons asked why the police were coming to the door at dinner time [after Gallo suggested to police that Crewdson might have broken into his house]. And he knew it from the rumors he kept catalogued in a file at home. Only one of those, he says, truly bothered him, because it reflected on his family. It was that Crewdson had divorced his wife to join a gay commune in San Francisco and had then "set up housekeeping with his boyfriends" in Bethesda. Though it was unclear if this tale, like the others, had originated with Gallo, Gallo had often tried to label his critics in AIDS as being gay; the story seemed to bear his stamp.

"I've caused problems for other people in my career," says Crewdson, understating the damage he helped unleash upon the Nixon White House, the FBI and the CIA, all of which were known to retaliate against journalists for less. "But I don't ever remember a government official engaging in a sustained personal attack on me or any other reporter." That Gallo is a physician, sworn to compassion, seems to make the situation all the more unusual.

—Barry Werth, "By AIDS Obsessed," *GQ*, August, 1991

"Gallo was certainly committing open and blatant scientific fraud," Sonnabend says. "But the point is not to focus on Gallo. It's us—all of us in the scientific community, we let him get away with it. None of this was hidden. It was all out in the open but nobody would say a word against Gallo. It had a lot to do with patriotism—the idea that this great discovery was made by an American."

—Celia Farber, "Fatal Distraction," *Spin*, June 1992

Robert Gallo was a sine qua non of what should be called "Holocaust II." It is unimaginable without him at the very core of its deadly insanity. He wasn't just a run-of-the-mill scientific villain. He was larger than life, someone you would expect to see in a Batman movie. One where Batman dies. The world owes a great debt of gratitude to John Crewdson, the

Pulitzer Prize winning *Chicago Tribune* journalist who mastered the irritating minutiae of retrovirology (and pseudoretrovirology) in order to capture Gallo in all of his exasperating and pathological glory.

In *Science Fictions*, the underappreciated book of microscopic reporting, John Crewdson piles up detail after detail of Gallo's career like a skilled novelist, determined to sear Gallo's essence into our consciousness and to leave us in a state of shock about what actually took place behind trusted laboratory doors while people were dying horrific deaths from AIDS all over the world. When Crewdson is done with his awesome dissection of Gallo, and we have seen the innards of the world's most amazing pathological liar laid out on the autopsy table, no reasonable observer should take *anything* Gallo said about AIDS seriously. Yet Crewdson himself seems to have ultimately had no qualms about leaving Gallo's theory that HIV causes AIDS standing totally hegemonic and unchallenged amid all the shocking evidence of Gallo's chronic incompetence and perfidiousness. It's a real puzzlement.

According to Crewdson, the early career of Robert C. Gallo, the world's most famous AIDS researcher at the National Cancer Institute, got off to a precocious start as a lab chief at the age of twenty-seven. But it was subsequently unsuccessful and frustrated until Gallo accomplished what appeared to some scientists at the time to have been his first viral theft. That may have involved stealing credit from the Japanese who discovered a virus named ATLV by renaming the same virus HTLV. Regardless of whether Gallo did steal credit for *that* virus, the questionable fog of its discovery certainly fit the funky pattern of what occurred in his lab during the 1980s when Gallo sank his teeth into the search for the cause of AIDS. And even beyond that. Crewdson establishes early in his lengthy book that Gallo is a man of great manipulative shtick. Gallo's mythological song and dance about himself and his origins is a somewhat revealing Dickensian story about the source of his professional drive and his great destiny: Crewdson writes, "In newspaper and magazine articles, Gallo's single-mindedness was frequently attributed to the death of his five-year old sister, Judith from childhood leukemia, an event Gallo recalled as the most traumatic of his young life, and which had transformed the Gallo household into a grim and joyless place without music or laughter where Thanksgiving and Christmas was no longer observed." (*SF* p.15) How could anyone question a man of such noble motives? (Actually, how could anyone *not*?)

In *Science Fictions*, Crewdson presents a Gallo who is a loud, crass braggart who people either loved in a toadying manner or, if they were streetwise, considered him to be what one scientist once described as a "black hole" that destroyed everything in its vicinity. Crewdson describes a period of early disgrace at the NCI during which Gallo had supposedly discovered the first evidence of reverse transcriptase "in human leukemia cells" which subsequently turned out to be irreproducible when another scientist tried to replicate the finding. (*SF* p.14) Bad luck struck again when Gallo was celebrated on the front page of *The Washington Post* only to have his discovery, a virus called HL23, undermined by one of his enemies who proved that what Gallo had was not a human retrovirus "but a melange of three animal viruses—a woolly monkey virus, a gibbon ape virus and a baboon virus—jumbled together in a retroviral cocktail." (*SF* p.19) A humiliating retraction was made subsequently in *Nature*. Unfortunately, this kind of failure in the life of a character like Gallo only made the man *more* determined to vindicate himself at all costs as a great scientist. The whole world would pay a terrible price for his extraordinary determination.

There is something about Robert Gallo—if you've ever met him in person or seen him on television or talked to him on the phone—that makes you wonder what planet or species he is from. Crewdson captures his uncanny strangeness when he notes, "Gallo's conversations often sounded as though a tape recording were being played back at faster than normal speed, and his syntax frequently lent the impression of someone whose first language was not English." (*SF* p.19) By the time Crewdson is done with him 600 pages later, one is convinced that Gallo's first language is falsehood.

Crewdson presents Gallo's lab in its early days as a place where things were *always mysteriously going wrong*. It wasn't just that the scientific findings the lab produced couldn't be replicated, but there were also odd break-ins and very peculiar acts of sabotage. But the best was yet to come.

Unfortunately, as Gallo's desperation for a big discovery grew, so had the budget of the National Cancer Institute as the nation committed itself to the desperate hunt for the viral origins of cancer. Richard Nixon cancer initiative was the wind beneath Gallo's wings. However, things got off to a disappointing start for many years and, in a moment of political bad timing, Gallo's HL23 scientific embarrassment happened shortly after there had already been numerous viral dead ends at NCI and the whole program was losing its luster and in real jeopardy of being cut back.

That the HL23 virus turned out to be a laboratory contaminant rather than a new virus *after it had been touted in the press*, even before its publication in a scientific journal became a familiar pattern in Gallo's scientific lifestyle (and may have been adopted by some of his underlings). Also to be repeated throughout his career was his inability to admit he was wrong about this HL23 until it couldn't seriously be denied. (*SF* p.19) The fact that the contaminant looked like it had to have been a deliberate act of sabotage by somebody suggested that even darker things were going on at the National Cancer Institute around Gallo, things that even ubersleuth John Crewdson may have been unable to nail down. This dark possibility of an *even bigger missed story* is a cloud that hovers over all the events in Crewdson's narrative.

According to Crewdson, the only reason that Gallo's career didn't go down the tubes over the HL23 debacle was because he had a protector at NCI, his boss Vincent DeVita, someone who would come to Gallo's rescue more than once during his troubled tenure at the Institute. (*SF* p.20) Crewdson writes that DeVita was one of a number of people who held the opinion that Gallo was basically a genius who was also a handful. This was a tragic flaw in DeVita's judgment that would have terrible consequences for the legacy of American biomedical science and the health of every person on this planet.

Crewdson portrays Gallo as a man rabidly obsessed with winning a Nobel Prize (*SF* p.20) He was ready to do whatever needed to be done and to elbow out everyone who got in his way. He had no qualms about cheating his subordinates out of appropriate credit for their (sometimes questionable) discoveries. He was also happy to reward achievement of subordinates by unceremoniously getting rid of them when they threatened to outshine him. (*SF* p.23) Gallo's bizarre, paranoid laboratory was the object of suspicion from other scientific quarters. When his lab supposedly discovered HTLV, Gallo refused to let samples of that virus leave his lab and Crewdson quotes a colleague of Gallo's as saying there was "a feeling around the N.I.H. that there was something, ah, wrong with HTLV." (*SF* p.31) Gallo may have realized early in his career that if you didn't want people to find anything wrong with your work the best thing to do is to *not share your viruses—or anything else—with them.*

The funny thing about Gallo, surely one of the most paranoid people to ever call himself a scientist, is that he was always accusing *others* of paranoia and baseless suspicion—toward him and his eminently questionable motives. When it seemed to some scientists that Gallo's lab had switched the Japanese virus, ATLV, with the Gallo lab's supposed version of the same virus (the soon-to-be celebrated HTLV), he argued that it was paranoid for anyone to even dare to think that way. (*SF* p.32) For

Gallo, there was always something structurally wrong with the brains of the people who witnessed his crimes. They were always crazy, and he was always sane. You could say that Gallo was from the blame-the-victim-school of scientific fraud.

Adding insult to injury, after what looked like a viral theft of ATLV from the Japanese, he barely gave them any credit at all for their research into the very virus his lab seems to have taken advantage of. And he mocked the work of the Japanese on ATLV several times (*SF* p.36) The Crewdson picture of Gallo throughout the book is of a man with absolutely no shame.

Two of Gallo's subordinates, the so-called hands-on discoverers of the suspiciously discovered HTLV, Bernard Poiesz and Francis Ruscetti, got the usual treatment that putatively successful people (or co-virus-lifters) got in Gallo's lab. Ruscetti went on "the endangered list" and was never cited in the award Gallo was given for the discovery of HTLV. Poiesz was betrayed by Gallo in the form of receiving a lukewarm endorsement from Gallo when he applied for a grant. Crewdson quotes Poiesz as saying about Gallo's credit-grab for the discovery of HTLV that it was "like saying that Queen Isabella discovered America after Columbus came home told her about it." (*SF* p.37)

Unfortunately, in terms of the world's biomedical safety, Gallo was in the wrong place at the wrong time when AIDS occurred and initially he had the wrong virus at the ready: HTLV, of course, because that's what he happened to be working on. Just the adoption of the idea that HTLV might be the cause of AIDS (an idea supposedly given to Gallo by others) was patently absurd and raises questions about Gallo's scientific judgment. It may have been purely driven by the prurient fact that the Japanese, according to Crewdson, "had shown that HTLV was transmitted by sexual intercourse." (*SF* p.39) The fact that the CDC had given him a gay-obsessed and sexual epidemiological paradigm to work with didn't help matters. One feels a sense of dread at the prospect of Gallo getting involved in anything with a sexual angle when Crewdson quotes the CDC's Cy Cabradillo talking about Gallo: "He [Gallo] didn't seem that interested. . . . I don't think he wanted to get involved with a gay disease. What turned him around was Max [Essex]." (*SF* p. 41) One almost wishes that Gallo's homophobia or gay-antipathy had been even more pronounced and that Essex had weaker powers of persuasion and that Gallo had blown off requests to get involved in AIDS. It would have saved the gay community and the rest of the world from decades of grief.

What was so intellectually challenged about Gallo's notion that HTLV could even remotely be the cause of AIDS was the fact that, as most retrovirologists knew, "quite apart from killing T-cells," HTLV "transformed them into leukemic cells." (*SF* p.44) But that didn't stop Gallo once it became his idée fixe. Gallo was always light-years ahead of his data—imaginary and real.

While Gallo was promoting the silly notion that HTLV was the cause of AIDS, French researchers at the Pasteur Institute in Paris discovered a retrovirus they called "LAV" in the lymph nodes of AIDS patients. Gallo pulled off one of his many fast ones when he offered to submit Pasteur's LAV paper on the discovery to *Science*. When they took him up on the offer, he noticed the Pasteur scientists had failed to write an abstract, in a moment of fake generosity he called Luc Montagnier and said he would be willing to write the abstract (*SF* p.56) One should always beware of Gallos bearing gifts. According to Crewdson, "To his everlasting regret, Montagnier agreed." (*SF* p.56) What Crewdson described at this early point in his account of Gallo is so egregiously crooked that it boggles the mind that anyone subsequently ever took at face value *any of the science* that came out of that NCI den of biomedical iniquity. Gallo completely distorted the meaning of the Pasteur paper in the abstract he concocted, an intellectual act of dishonesty so in-your-face that it takes one's breath away. In the true spirit of the opposite world of abnormal science, Gallo twisted the whole meaning of the Pasteur paper to point towards his own birdbrained notion that *their AIDS related virus was actually HTLV*. According to Crewdson, "As summarized by Gallo . . . the French manuscript appeared to be reporting, if not the isolation of HTLV itself, then a very closely related virus." (*SF* p.56) And to add humor to injury, Gallo ran the abstract by the French on the phone, reading it so quickly that, according to Crewdson, they didn't even understand it. It didn't stop there. Robert Gallo also altered some of the text of the French paper, again in the direction of making it sound like the French retrovirus was from the same viral family as his own misguided HTLV. Montagnier had deliberately called it a "lymphotropic virus" to make sure it was *not* confused with the members of the HTLV family. Montagnier criticized Gallo's obsession with HTLV, insisting "Gallo didn't believe there could be more than one kind of human retrovirus. He was fully convinced that HTLV was the right one, that there was only one human retrovirus involved in AIDS." (*SF* p.57) As was typical in the self-dealing abnormal, totalitarian science of AIDS, the reviewer for the paper turned out to be the paper's re-writer himself, Robert Gallo. Not surprisingly, he gave the French paper that he himself altered "his enthusiastic endorsement." (*SF* p.57) And for good measure he basically misled again in his letter to *Science* with the paper, telling the editor that Montagnier agreed with it all. (*SF* p.57)

Curiously, in terms of the role of HHV-6 in AIDS, Crewdson notes the fact that at that point Gallo's boss, Vince DeVita, thought that HTLV, the virus Gallo was pushing, was actually *a passenger virus*. De Vita may have been a true visionary.

Gallo's HTLV baloney gained credibility when his Harvard pal, Myron Essex, published a very questionable report that "between a quarter and a third of the AIDS patients he tested had antibodies to HTLV." (*SF* p.58) The publication made Essex an instant millionaire the day after its publication because Essex owned stock in a company that manufactured tests for HTLV, the virus that ultimately would turn out to have nothing to do with AIDS. (*SF* p.58) He wasn't the only one to get rich peddling bogus science during "Holocaust II."

What could have been a cautionary note about the herd-of-sheep psyche of the abnormal, totalitarian world of AIDS research in general can be found in Crewdson's amusing passage about other scientists' ostrich-like inattention to the total lack of logic in blaming a leukemia causing virus for a disease that involved the killing of t-cells. Instead of questioning Gallo and Essex's bizarre HTLV logic, according to Crewdson, potential critics and people who should have known better *doubted themselves*. They had been successfully gaslighted. He quotes one of the deferential self-doubters: "'I didn't consider myself capable of questioning Max Essex,' one researcher recalled. 'Max Essex was a person at Harvard. That meant that Max Essex would probably be right. The likelihood that he needed me to re-evaluate his data was zero.'" (*SF* p.59) This was Myron "FOCMA" Essex he was talking about. In the abnormal scientific community of AIDS research your data wasn't the issue. The school you were associated with was all that mattered. (If historians ever wake up and there is any justice in the world, one day, thanks to Essex, the word "Harvard" will be a synonymous with scientific fraud. Maybe one day it will be even used as a verb, as in "to Harvard the data" or "to Harvard the books.")

Much like Gallo, Essex usually had a reason why he was always right and others were always wrong. According to Crewdson, "asked why *if* [HTLV] was the cause of AIDS, he had only found antibodies in fewer than half the AIDS patients he tested, Essex replied that his test probably wasn't sensitive enough." (*SF* p.59) When Gallo was asked the same question about his own study that found HTLV in only four of three dozen AIDS patients Crewdson notes, "Gallo suggested that the virus was difficult to find when the number of remaining T-cells was small." (*SF* p.59) And Crewdson reports that Gallo even had a Galloesque answer for why there was virtually no AIDS in Japan where there was a great deal of HTLV: "Gallo replied that AIDS simply hadn't been noticed in Japan or maybe the Japanese responded differently to HTLV than Africans or Americans." (*SF* p.59)

Gallo's prestidigitations were very successful at making the media and the public think the French researchers were barking up the same HTLV retroviral tree he was. He highhandedly went so far as to suggest the French should actually *stop working* on their virus if it wasn't the same as HTLV. And Gallo did everything he could do to encourage other scientists not to take the French discovery seriously. Crewdson artfully captures Gallo constantly talking out of both sides of mouth about the relationship—or lack of one—between the French virus and his beloved HTLV. Crewdson reports that Gallo's own staff *had in fact* done the necessary research to determine that they were different viruses and according to Crewdson, "Whatever Gallo was saying in public, in private he agreed with his staff." (*SF* p.63) One could always count on there being two sets of books in the abnormal science of AIDS, especially in Gallo's laboratory.

The French were in a vulnerable position where Gallo was concerned because, according to Crewdson, they were afraid that he might cut off their access to scientific publication. (*SF* p.71) Gallo was a serious power broker in the world of science and that certainly should have been more of a warning sign to the scientific community that the very essence of AIDS science was mired in questionable hardball politics. Gallo even had enough power to be able to threaten the Centers for Disease Control. When the CDC dared to complain that Gallo was not sharing his HTLV probes, according to Crewdson, Gallo sniffily threatened to not cooperate with the organization. (*SF* p.74) "There was a fight," one scientist told Crewdson, "between the CDC and Gallo over who was supposed to be gathering data from research. Gallo felt they should be gathering data, and he should be doing the science." (*SF* p.74) Whatever that means. Gallo didn't realize what a perfect match his kind of virology actually made for the CDC's kind of epidemiology. Scientifically speaking, it was like the mafia families of two major cities joining forces.

One crossed Gallo at one's great peril. According to Crewdson, when a scientist named David Purtillo began to find serious evidence that *not a single*

AIDS patient in his study was positive for HTLV, he found that *Science* magazine "wasn't interested in undercutting its high-visibility articles." (*SF* p.75) When Joseph Sonnabend, a New York AIDS doctor who was the first editor of *AIDS Research*, a small journal, dared to publish the Gallo-challenging Purtillo findings, according to Crewdson, "the publisher of *AIDS Research* replaced Sonnabend with [Gallo crony] Dani Bolognesi, who promptly installed Gallo on the journal's editorial board." (*SF* p.75) That's how scientific publishing worked during "Holocaust II." You scratch *my* back and I'll destroy *your* enemies.

As evidence piled up showing that the French had found the so-called AIDS retrovirus, Gallo imperiously dug in his heels for his HTLV. So did his Harvard pal Myron Essex who had spent his formative years with his buddy Gallo just trying to convince the scientific community that retroviruses *do* really cause cancer. Together they did their best to dampen the world's enthusiasm for the French virus as the probable cause of AIDS. It was one of the great examples of teamwork in science.

Gallo saw his HTLV dream start to fade when Montagnier showed up at a scientific meeting that was focused on Gallo's own candidate for AIDS virus. Montagnier presented evidence that patients who were positive for the French retrovirus were *not* positive for Gallo's HTLV. (*SF* p.81) And even worse, according to Crewdson, he "pointed out the similarities between LAV and the Equine Infectious Anemia Virus rather than HTLV." (*SF* p.81) And most threatening of all to Gallo's dreams of a Nobel Prize was the fact that Montagnier had found LAV in "63 percent of pre-AIDS patients and 20 percent of those with AIDS but less than 2 percent of the general population." (*SF* p.81) At the meeting at which Montagnier made his dramatic presentation, Crewdson wrote that Gallo did his best to cast aspersions on the research, bizarrely "questioning the reality of the reverse transcriptase activity." (*SF* p.81) According to one scientist at the meeting who is quoted by Crewdson, "[Gallo] insulted Montagnier. It was a disgusting display, absolutely disgusting. He told him it was terrible science, that there was no way it could be true. He ranted and raved for eight or ten minutes." (*SF* p.81) And of course, while Gallo was publicly humiliating Montagnier, *privately* he was asking for more samples of the French virus. (*SF* p.81)

The French discovery made it clear that Gallo had led the whole scientific community into a retroviral cul-de-sac, but at a later conference in Paris, he was at it again, playing the same tiresome duplicitous game, pushing bogus HTLV while evidence was clearly accumulating against it.

Gallo could feign and bully like nobody else in the history of science. One scientist described to Crewdson a fight Gallo had with Montagnier: "During that fight one had the impression Montagnier was a little boy and Gallo was a genius. Because Montagnier didn't argue well." (*SF* p.87) Gallo wore his opposition down with over-the-top verbal displays. The word "bully" comes to mind.

Gallo changed gears from the deadender HTLV to a virus that he could get away with calling the cause of AIDS the old fashioned way: he stole it. The complicated manner in which that was obfuscated and outrageously covered up makes up the main investigative feast in Crewdson's book. Gallo's decade of gymnastic AIDS mendacities might have been lost to history without the laser vision and crystal clear exposition of John Crewdson. If not for *New York Native* and John "Javert" Crewdson, Gallo would have gotten away with murder. Make that "genocide."

Even when Gallo's lab was pursuing a new virus like the one the French had, Gallo kept up the public pretense that HTLV was the very best candidate for the cause of AIDS. His laboratory was secretly and frantically playing a game of catch-up with the French. They had received samples of the French virus and were not honest about what they were doing with them. Gallo's subordinates privately confirmed that the French virus could be found in AIDS patients, but it would never be admitted publicly. Adding insult to deception, because Gallo had so polluted the scientific community with his stubborn, delusional notion that HTLV had to be the only possible cause, the French had trouble getting their growing body of research on LAV published. *Science* turned down an important paper that made it clear once and for all that the French LAV was not the Gallo HTLV. (*SF* p. 98) Gallo was dismissing their discovery with one hand and appropriating it with the other.

At a conference in Park City, Utah in late 1983, Gallo played his familiar game of asking disingenuous and disparaging questions publicly after a Pasteur presentation on LAV. Meanwhile, Gallo ignored doubts about his own HTLV by scientists like Jay Levy, "who wanted to know why, if HTLV caused AIDS, AIDS patients didn't have T-cell leukemia." (*SF* p.99) According to Crewdson, the obdurate Dr. Gallo insisted to Levy that "HTLV itself . . . *could* still cause AIDS." (*SF* p.99)

Luckily for the French, scientists at the CDC, home of the "impeccable" original AIDS nosology and epidemiology, had growing doubts themselves about HTLV, and even Myron Essex's old protégé, AIDS researcher and retrovirus aficionado, Donald Francis, was ready to jump ship. Crewdson captures one of many ironic moments in "Holocaust II" when he quotes Don Francis as saying, "It had become clear . . . that we had made a very big mistake." (*SF* p.100) Unfortunately, Francis didn't have a clue that he and his associates at the CDC and NIH were about to make an *exponentially even bigger virological mistake* that would threaten the whole world's health.

Thanks to the fact that his staff was working with the retrovirus foolishly supplied by the gullible French scientists, Gallo was finally seeing some interesting numbers of AIDS patients testing positive—and given what he was working with why wouldn't he? After he developed his own blood test for his purloined retrovirus, the CDC tried to determine if the French or Gallo had the best test for detecting an AIDS case. The Pasteur test did slightly better in a competition between the two country's tests and lest things be done on the up and up, according to Crewdson, Gallo wanted the CDC to *alter the results* so as to reflect a better score for Gallo's version of the test—another typical moment in the abnormal, totalitarian, and sociopathic science of "Holocaust II." To his eternal discredit, Jim Curran, the top AIDS researcher at the CDC, *actually agreed to Gallo's ridiculous request to alter the results.* To do otherwise would have been to commit normal science. Giving Gallo that unholy advantage was just one more enabling act that helped Gallo become the top spokesman for the infernal HIV/AIDS paradigm throughout "Holocaust II."

The minute that the CDC gave Gallo the word that his test for the so-called AIDS retrovirus was as good as the Pasteur one (or *sort of* as good), Gallo went into extreme Gallo mode, crowing to the world about his supposed achievement, and even more charmingly, according to Crewdson, he began "denigrating the work in Paris." (*SF* p.109) He told people he was "far ahead of the French." (*SF* p.109)

Gallo subsequently submitted data on his retroviral "discovery" in four papers to *Science*. The papers never said where the virus actually came from because they didn't dare. Mika Popovic, the unlucky scientist in Gallo's lab who did most of the bench work on the virus Gallo stole, watched as his manuscripts about the so-called discovery of the AIDS virus were methodically altered by Gallo. According to Crewdson, "entire sentences, even whole paragraphs had been excised, replaced with Gallo's scrawled additions. Crossed out altogether was the paragraph in which Popovic acknowledged the Pasteur's discovery of LAV and explained here that the French virus was 'described here' as HTLV-3." (*SF* p.111) From the scientific documents that would change the world forever, Gallo had taken out any acknowledgement of the Pasteur discovery. (*SF* p.111) In one of the most notorious notations of Gallo's whole wackadoodle career, next to a passage in which Popovic wrote something about LAV, Gallo scribbled, "Mika, are you crazy?" (*SF* p.111) Screamed the pot to the kettle.

One of the most important of the four seminal *Science* papers contained the egregious falsehood that Gallo's virus, which he called HTLV-3, had been isolated from 48 patients. Gallo also made sure, according to Crewdson, that the only reference to the French virus in the paper "sounded as though the French had the wrong virus." (*SF* p.111) Even though Gallo had basically used LAV to "discover" HTLV-3, he kept disingenuously insisting that LAV and HTLV-3 were different viruses. And even though the French had provided Gallo with LAV, and Gallo's staff knew all too well that they were not different in the least, Gallo lied to the French when they asked why he had not compared HTLV-3 to LAV and reported on it in the seminal science papers. One of Gallo's biggest lies to the French was "that Popovic hadn't been able to grow enough LAV to make comparisons." (*SF* p.118)

As Gallo was preparing to present the world premiere of the so-called virus that causes AIDS, he at first offered to include the French in the announcement to the world about the "discovery" of the virus and to cut the CDC—which had also played a role in the process—out of the deal. He then turned around and offered to make the announcement with the CDC and cut the French out of the deal. (*SF* p.119) Polyamory in the Gallo universe consisted of everyone having a chance to screw other people with Gallo before they themselves got screwed.

A sign of Gallo's enormous power in the intellectually challenged world of abnormal, totalitarian and sociopathic AIDS science was the fact that his "manuscripts were accepted by *Science* nineteen days after their submission." (*SF* p.123) A suggestion from *Science* that four papers were too many got the immediate Gallo threat that he could easily take his papers elsewhere. (*SF* p.123) The original papers had needed pictures of the virus that Gallo had supposedly discovered, and Gallo had them: they were pictures of the French virus relabeled as Gallo's HTLV-3. At least Gallo was consistent.

Crewdson's book doesn't just focus on the fact that Gallo's historic AIDS papers in *Science* were full of purloined credit he didn't deserve. In terms of the thesis that much of AIDS science was the work of pseudoscientific sloppiness, it is important to point out that Crewdson also wrote, "An astute reader might have noticed that Gallo's condition for labeling a virus HTLV-3 were so ambiguous that nearly any retrovirus, animal, or human, would have qualified." (*SF* p.124) In the opposite world of abnormal science here are no rules to keep science from becoming a big Alice-in-Wonderland mess. About the original papers Crewdson said something that only increased the irony and tragedy of Crewdson ultimately himself accepting the HIV/AIDS paradigm: ". . . a perceptive reviewer might even have questioned Gallo's claim to have found the presumptive cause of AIDS." (*SF* p.124) (If only Crewdson had jumped in for the sake of the whole world and done with his acute journalistic skills what a perceptive reviewer *should* have done. Tragically, two frauds were passing in the night.)

A strange incident occurred just prior to the publication of the big four papers in *Science*, one that captures Gallo in all his zany treacherousness. Gallo had voluntarily given a European reporter copies of his forthcoming *Science* papers, and when the reporter published a story about them—under the reasonable impression that he wasn't breaking any embargo—Gallo accused the reporter "of having stolen the four *Science* manuscripts from his office while Gallo's back was turned." (*SF* p.126)

The theft of the French virus was not just a theft of credit from the French. It was also a theft of money in the form of lost royalties for the tests that would be developed from the purloined virus thought to be the cause of AIDS. Gallo's lab had essentially pulled off an unarmed scientific robbery; the French were destined by Gallo's shenanigans to lose millions of dollars. The matter was made even ethically worse (if the virus actually was the true cause of AIDS) by the fact that the test Gallo's people developed using the stolen virus was inferior to the test developed by the Pasteur Institute. (*SF* p.128)

Some in the American government knew from the start that Gallo was pulling off a scientific heist. On the eve of the announcement by HHS Secretary Margaret Heckler, NIH Director Ed Brant received a phone call from James Curran and Donald Francis of the CDC warning him "that Heckler was about to make a huge mistake: the French, not Gallo, had been the first to find the cause of AIDS." (*SF* p.130) Unfortunately, the duplicitous train had left the station and the American government's scientific establishment was about to apply several layers of egg to its face. (And that didn't even involve the fact that the stolen, supposedly exogenous, retrovirus wasn't even the cause of AIDS.) During the April 23, 1984 announcement debacle, Gallo even went out of his way to make sure that absolutely *no credit* was given to the French for their role in the discovery. As if it wasn't absurd enough that the Secretary of HHS was celebrating a stolen discovery, she also confidently announced, "We hope to have . . . a vaccine ready for testing in about two years." (*SF* p. 135) She seems to have been off by, well, like forever.

The credulous media fell for the Gallo scam, generally downplaying the French contribution and the Pasteur scientists were appropriately apoplectic. Predictably, Gallo, according to Crewdson, "set about expunging the evidence that he had spent two years chasing the wrong virus. (*SF* p.144). Not only could Gallo do viral theft, but he was also one of science's greatest expungers and time travelers. He rewrote the remarks he had given at past scientific conferences to make it look like he was on the trail of the AIDS virus (which he called HTLV-3) all along when in actuality he had aggressively been pushing the lost cause, HTLV. In abnormal, totalitarian and sociopathic science the past is carved in sand.

After Gallo's big splash in *Science*, he often bragged about things that were not even in the papers, findings that had actually never even been accomplished in his lab. He also violated one of the collegial rules of science by refusing to share his viruses or cell lines with other scientists unless they agreed to certain bizarre and highly suspect preconditions. (*SF* p.149) According to Crewdson, for some scientists "Gallo tried to impose conditions on which experiments they could perform and which they could not." (*SF* p.149) Gallo forced one scientist to sign an agreement not to compare Gallo's virus to other viruses. (*SF* p.150) One either played by the rules of abnormal, totalitarian, and sociopathic science or one did not play at all. Gallo wanted to control what people said about his virus and who they shared it with. He knew what was at stake if the truth ever came out.

Even the powerful Centers for Disease Control could not get Gallo to cooperate by sharing his cell lines. When noises started to be made in Paris and down in Atlanta at the CDC that Gallo had not really discovered the "AIDS retrovirus," Gallo went grandiosely ballistic, saying strange things like "We started the field. We predicted AIDS." (*SF* p.153) Like a Donald Trump of science, he accused anyone who tried to tell the truth about the matter of spreading "plot and innuendo." (*SF* p.156) The husband of Flossie Wong-Stahl, a woman who worked closely (actually, more than closely) with Gallo in his lab astutely described Gallo and his milieu to Crewdson: "The whole business has the ethics of a used-car lot. It's what you can get away with. The older-style scientists are falling by the wayside. To be a success in science these days, you need a big operation. . . . It's become an entrepreneurial business and Gallo's good at that . . . He was one of the first big-time laboratory operators." (*SF* p.158) One could say that "Holocaust II" was partly born in a used-car lot in which nobody was allowed to kick the tires.

The world fell easily for Robert Gallo, his stolen virus, and his very questionable science. According to Crewdson, Gallo received a major honor from "the Italian-American Foundation . . . that compared Gallo to Galileo." (*SF* p.158) Lysenko would have been a more appropriate comparison. If that wasn't enough, both his boss and the future Director of the NIH would compare him to Mozart. To the rest of the world he would be the great man who had discovered the cause of AIDS. You could say it was the triumph of Salieri.

When his luck did start to change and people spoke more openly and brazenly about Gallo's virus-lifting, Gallo predictably tried to turn the tables and actually suggested that the French had made the mistake as a result of a contamination by *his* virus, which was patently ridiculous, as Crewdson shows in his book with detailed chronology of the actual events. All the evidence pointed to a contamination in Gallo's lab—at best. (*SF* p.162)

Unfortunately for the future scientific credibility of the American government, Crewdson points out, "The National Cancer Institute preferred Gallo's version of events." (*SF* p.162) It's interesting that the NIH uncharacteristically tried to silence Gallo when he actually may have been inadvertently trying to tell the truth about the nature of *the real epidemic*. Crewdson writes that the Director of NIH "tried to muzzle [Gallo]" when he "speculated publicly on the risk of transmitting AIDS to women via heterosexual contact." (*SF* p.163) But, Crewdson notes, "Gallo wouldn't stay quiet. After Jerry Groopman and Zaki Salahuddin reported detecting the AIDS virus in the saliva of nearly half of pre-AIDS patients, Gallo warned the American people that direct contact with saliva 'should be avoided,' setting off alarms about the safety of oral sex, water fountains, restaurant cutlery, and cardiopulmonary resuscitation." (*SF* p.163) That wasn't exactly how the government wanted to frame and promote the epidemiological image of the AIDS epidemic. Very interesting, in retrospect. Propaganda was about to control everything the world knew about AIDS.

Even after it was clear that HTLV-3 (as Gallo renamed LAV) was not a member of the HTLV family of retroviruses, Gallo stubbornly and perversely continued to aggressively promote the bogus notion. He even published data trying to fudge the issue. (*SF* p.163) And as could be expected, according to Crewdson, he continued his two-faced act: "Whatever Gallo was saying in print, in private he was far from certain that the AIDS virus had anything in common with the HTLVs." (*SF* p.163)

One of the more bizarre things about the so-called discovery of the AIDS virus in Gallo's lab was the fact that early on, according to Crewdson, "Gallo hadn't said a word about the patient in whom Popovic had found it." (*SF* p.164) It turned out that it hadn't even been found in an individual patient but it had "been isolated from the T-cells of several AIDS patients, whose cultured cells Popovic had pooled together." (*SF* p.164) As some scientists would say, WTF? As was typical of the kind of science and reporting that underlay the HIV/AIDS paradigm, this Frankenstein of a "patient pool" was not mentioned in the seminal, history-changing paper published in *Science*, the cornerstone of the HIV/AIDS paradigm. According to Crewdson, Donald Francis of the CDC "thought it odd still that Popovic had pooled patient material in the first place, something Francis viewed as a certain way not to know which patient was the source." (*SF* p.164) Not really knowing where a virus had come from was the characteristic way science was done in the opposite world of AIDS research. Assuming where things came from characterized the nosology, epidemiology and virology of AIDS.

Like many of Gallo's lies, the LAV lie was not without its dark humor. Not only was the virus Gallo worked with the same virus that the French had discovered, but most damning, *it even turned out originally to be from the exact same patient.* (*SF* p.165) A scientist named Murray Gardner confronted Gallo about this malarkey and according to Crewdson, Gardner said, "Bob browbeat me, in his way, for about an hour. . . . He questioned my patriotism, He asked me, 'Are you French or are you American? Aren't you an American?'" (*SF* p.167) If nothing else, the pseudoscience was patriotic.

At a time when Gallo should have been bathing in the glow of being the discoverer of the so-called AIDS virus, according to Crewdson, "Most of his energy was being devoted to fending off suspicions that his discovery was really somebody else's discovery." (*SF* p.177) It was becoming clearer to the world that "the virus discovered in Paris in 1983 was the same virus Gallo claimed to have discovered in 1984." (*SF* p.178)

Even after the discovery issue was on its way to being resolved in the favor of the French scientists, Gallo, without a single qualm, bizarrely insisted in retaining his HTLV-3 name for the virus. It mattered not to Gallo that the virus was obviously *not* a member of the HTLV family. And just as absurdly, he performed all kinds of silly mental acrobatics to try and explain why his virus was exactly like the French virus, suggesting that his virus came from someone who must have gotten infected at the same place and the same time as the French AIDS victim from whom the French had isolated their virus. You could call the mythic person Gallo's own "Patient Zero." According to Crewdson, "The French dismissed Gallo's explanation as balderdash. (*SF* p. 180)

What was it like to be a part of the Gallo team during those heady days when the French virus was stolen and the pseudoscientific foundation of "Holocaust II" was laid down? Omar Sattaur, a journalist who covered Gallo for the publication *New Scientist*, recounted to Crewdson that one of Gallo's subordinates told him "that everybody in Gallo's lab felt paranoid in some way and that it was quite an awful place to work. Because it was very high-pressure and he ran it like an autocrat. They were his minions." (*SF* p.183) Anybody who messed with Captain Hook walked the plank.

The *New Scientist* reporter was one of the first people to nail the details of the Gallo theft in print. The piece resulted in one of Gallo's biggest critics, Oxford scientist Abraham Karpas referring to the affair as "Gallogate." (*SF* p.184) Karpas was on the money in more ways than he ever realized. But the real "Gallogate" went way beyond the stealing of a retrovirus. Unbeknownst to Karpas and Sattaur, it was ultimately about something that would cause biomedical consequences for every member of the human race. Gallo's world class narcissism manifest itself in the fact that he told Sattaur that he was of a mind to have the government start a libel action against him. What is even more absurd is that given the government's bizarre (and not fully-fathomed in Crewdson's book) relationship with Gallo, one could almost imagine that actually happening. Omar Sattaur astutely captured the Gallo psyche when he said to Crewdson, "Gallo has this ability to just absorb everything . . . He's wonderful at it. He's so good at manipulating things that I'm pretty sure that unconsciously he's doing it most of the time. If you talk to him about other people's work, he'll say, 'Well, he worked in my lab for six weeks. I taught him everything he knew.' He's a real megalomaniac." (*SF* p.185) There was something uncanny about Gallo that, unfortunately, seemed to bemuse people at the same time that it disturbed them, so that even some of the most sober minds that came into his outrageous orbit somehow missed that fact that they were in the presence of a very unique kind of monster, a human whose actions and statements, from his victim's and history's point of view, heralded from a psychic netherworld located somewhere in the vortex of clownishness, sociopathology and downright evil. One can't help but speculate that because the marginalized people whose lives hung in the balance were "gay,"—or "very gay," as the CDC's James Curran would say—that extreme moral outrage on the part of most heterosexual scientists (and some gay ones too, unfortunately) often took a vacation in Gallo's presence. Gallo wasn't playing his infernal games with breast cancer, prostate cancer, or heart disease. No matter what lip service people gave to broaden the perceived social spectrum of this particular disease, from the extant scientific community's perspective (and the public's) *it was gay through and through*.

As previously pointed out, Gallo's crime against the French was not just the intangible one of falsely claiming primacy of discovery. The theft was also a major financial crime in that he was also stealing the Pasteur's rightful royalties from the test for the so-called AIDS retrovirus. The American government's patents had all been hurriedly filed under the false pretenses that Gallo had created them with a virus that he had actually discovered. And to make matters even crazier, in terms of testing for the retrovirus virus that was now considered to be the cause of AIDS, his fraud-based test *didn't even work as well as the French test*. (*SF*. p.188) Gallo's rushed filing for the AIDS test patent, according to Crewdson, "had been approved in near-record time," (*SF* p.191) another dramatic indication that the government was in bed with Gallo. Crewdson reported, "The French application had fallen between the cracks, and nobody at the patent office seemed to have noticed." (*SF* p.192)

One of the zanier details of the Gallo biography is the fact that he had a baby with one of the married scientists who worked with him, Flossie-Wong Stahl, which was awkward for the rest of his staff—and for Wong-Stahl's husband. According to Crewdson, the messy affair resulted in Gallo "being put in the hands of a psychiatrist for a while." (*SF* p.194) In terms of Gallo's impact on the world, it may be a shame that it was only for "a while." (The catastrophic HHV-6 pandemic might have been nipped in the bud if the whole Gallo lab had been put in the hands of a psychiatrist.)

When journalists all over the world started to wake up to the fact that Gallo had stolen credit for discovering the AIDS virus, Gallo became a whirling dervish. One science reporter told Crewdson, "Bob Gallo would write to every journalist in the world who would publish an article that wouldn't be completely in favor with his point of view. He would explode. He would immediately conclude that the journalist who had written the article that was not in favor of his genius was prejudiced, was poorly informed, was a friend of Pasteur or something like that." (*SF* p.196) He could have taught Donald Trump a trick or two.

Ever proactive, Gallo went to Paris and got Jean Claude Chermann, (one of the members of the Pasteur's LAV team) drunk and had him sign a phony, Gallo-friendly rewrite of the history of the discovery of the so-called AIDS virus. (*SF* p.198) According to Crewdson, "Gallo promised the document would never see the light of the day. Back in the United States, however, Gallo sent a copy to Jim Weingarten [the Director of NIH]." (*SF* p.198) And when the incorrigible Gallo sent documents to a French journalist in order to bolster his claims that he had not stolen the virus from the French, he included an old letter from Chermann which had been doctored in classic Gallo style. Chermann happened to see the doctored letter and according to Crewdson, "When Chermann compared the letter sent by Gallo to the original in his files, he saw that someone had cut out his signature and posted it at the end of the third paragraph, transforming what had been a scathing two-page critique of Gallo's behavior into a one-page testimonial. (*SF* p.199) This is not exactly what Thomas Kuhn would call "normal science."

It will forever be a dark blemish on the integrity of the top people in the American government's scientific establishment that the Health and Human Services elite went to bat for this scientific shyster. The Pasteur Institute could not believe the institutional support that the Gallo was getting, but now they were not about to be intimidated. They were ready to sue their way to the truth about the discovery in the American courts and to secure their just rewards from the AIDS test patent. What is really disturbing in the Crewdson account of the affair is that the government gradually *did* start to realize that Gallo's discovery claim was bogus, but the authorities shamefully continued to bolster Gallo's defense. And, in keeping with the Gallo habit of leaving no supportive deed unpunished, he turned around and blamed the American government itself for filing the patent that had enriched him and had enhanced his reputation. Even more outrageous was the fact that he was telling people that he made no money from the patent, about which one government official said to Crewdson, "Well I didn't see him turn his checks down when they came to him." (*SF* p.204) According to Crewdson, " . . . with the AIDS test earning millions— both Gallo and Popovic qualified for the maximum payment—$100,000 a year during the lifetime of the patent, a total of $1.5 million apiece over fifteen years. The AIDS test had made them millionaires."(*SF* p.278) Some of the biggest beneficiaries of AIDS fraud would be Gallo's favorite restaurants.

One of the most stunning revelations in Crewdson's book, as we have already pointed out, is that Gallo's lab wasn't just mendacious, but at the same time it also seems to have been surprisingly sloppy and disorganized which is exactly what one wants to hear about the place that helped lay down the foundation of the AIDS paradigm. The Pasteur Institute, on the other hand, (at least on the surface) seems to have been a model of fastidiousness. Crewdson describes their record keeping: "Pasteur scientists kept the records of their experiments in the European style, in sequential hardbound volumes that made it impossible to insert or remove pages of what had transpired in their labs." (*SF* p.206) In the opposite world of Gallo's lab, Mika Popovic, who did much of the work on the discovery or rediscovery of the AIDS virus "didn't have any notebooks." (*SF* p.206) Gallo is quoted as saying, about Popovic's record keeping, "We were finding stuff in drawers, pieces of paper . . . I mean we pulled out stuff that Mika didn't even know he had. And there it was. You know, old stuff, old archaic papers with scribbles on them." (*SF* p.206) Crewdson reported that "the scraps proved to be the only records Popovic could produce of what the government now counted a landmark achievement." (*SF* p.206) Given what the landmark "achievement" would actually turn out to be, it shouldn't surprise anyone that it was arrived at in such a ramshackle "scientific" style. Popovic was quite generous with his scraps of paper once under investigation. According to Crewdson, when investigators came to look at his records he said, "Take whatever I have. I don't want to go to jail." (*SF* p.207)

It was convenient for Popovic's records to be that sloppy because the Humpty-Dumpty pieces of evidence almost made it impossible to reconstruct a credible narrative of exactly how Gallo had succeeded in using the French virus to pretend he had discovered his own. (Lesson to fraudulent scientists everywhere: sloppiness creates fabulous plausible deniability.) But Crewdson, the master detective, worked his way patiently though the devious trails of disorganized paper to make Gallo's theft of credit for the discovery painfully obvious. In the process, Crewdson found evidence that Gallo altered memos to reflect fraudulent dates for when important experiments were done. (*SF* p.208)

Gallo stonewalled when Health and Human Services tried to find out what happened in his laboratory in order to put together a defense for Gallo's claims in court. As Gallo tried to rewrite the past, Crewdson reports that all kinds of discrepancies emerged. There was a clear record that he had been pursuing HTLV-1 as the cause in the period that he now was disingenuously trying to convince the world that he was actually pursuing HTLV-3, which of course turned out to be the LAV which the French had provided his lab with.

The Perry Mason smoking gun moment that destroyed Gallo's credibility for all eternity came when it was discovered that the so-called AIDS virus was incredibly *changeable* and every isolate was dramatically different from every other isolate. When it was discovered that there was virtually *no difference* between Gallo's isolate of HTLV-3 and the French isolate of LAV, it was obvious that Gallo had indeed been working with the Pasteur's isolate, not an isolate that he had discovered.

As Gallo's luck would have it, his test for the AIDS virus, which was based on the stolen French virus, was not very reliable. The French test was supposedly much better but the Gallo test had won the licensing race politically and was often failing to detect blood that was supposedly infected. Gallo's test not only had a high rate of false negatives, but it also had false positives. Gallo's incompetent test ended up ruining a number of people's lives. (*SF* p. 228) (Of course the real problem with the testing for the retrovirus by either the French or American test was that it begged the larger theoretical question of whether either test was really the test for the true cause of so-called AIDS.)

Gallo exceeded his usual standard for craziness in the fight over the name of the virus he had stolen from the French. How dare the French want to name the virus they discovered! According to Crewdson, "When Gallo discovered the French were using the term LAV alone, he sent Montagnier a peevish letter." (*SF* p. 235) In the end the French were only half-screwed when the Gallo name of HTLV-3 did not prevail and the virus was labeled "Human immunodeficiency virus or HIV." (*SF* p.236) The fact that the new name was a kind of Orwellian way of disingenuously establishing that the virus was the cause of AIDS without the inconvenience of further debate was lost on most people. The lesson of this episode of abnormal, totalitarian, and sociopathic science is that if you want to prove that a virus is the cause of a disease, just *give it a name that implies that it is the cause*. With "Human immunodeficiency virus or HIV" that mission was brilliantly accomplished. A fun bit of trivia about the voting on the name change is that the only person to support Gallo's preference of HTLV-3 was—guess who?—Myron Essex. (*SF.* p.236) (The name of the virus was "Harvarded" into history.)

One of the most embarrassing moments in the Gallo affair was the point at which it was discovered that the photographs that Gallo's lab had submitted to *Science* which were identified as photos of *their* virus turned out to actually be photos of the French virus. According to Crewdson, "the revelation dealt a major blow to the [National Cancer Institute's] credibility.

(*SF* p.240) Gallo himself had a copy of the photo of the purloined virus in a framed collage on his office wall and Crewdson reports, "When Gallo found out the virus in the collage was LAV, Salahuddin [his subordinate] recalled 'he took it down from the wall and threw it on the floor, smashing glass everywhere.'" (*SF* p.241) One can only assume that like every other Gallo mess, someone else in his lab cleaned it up. The fake photo caper was one of the things that, according to Crewdson, helped turn Gallo's NCI boss, Vince DeVita, against him. Crewdson wrote, "DeVita was determined that Gallo would correct the record." (*SF* p.241)

What is mind-boggling about Gallo is that even while under investigation for the LAV fraud, he and his staff still continued to churn out *more* fraud. A letter from the Gallo folks published in *Nature* in May of 1986, meant to exonerate Gallo, contained brand new fibs. Gallo claimed to have isolated HTLV-3 from a patient he hadn't even been looking for the virus in at the time that was clearly impossible because it was the same period in which all the evidence showed he was still obsessed with HTLV-1. Gallo reconstructed a fictional past in the letter and included a picture that had just happened to have both HTLV-1 and LAV/HTLV-3 in it. According to Crewdson, he pretended to have discovered HTLV-3 earlier than he really did just by the happenstance of it being in the same photo. (*SF* p.244) One could call it a classic Gallo scientific discovery. Once again it was as if Gallo had a time machine that allowed him to go back into the past and fashion history more to his liking. Crewdson describes NCI scientist Berge Hampar's reaction to the new photo caper that appeared in *Nature*: "'When we saw *Nature*, we laughed,' Hampar said. 'We said, "Is this the only photograph they got? They're staking all their claims on one photograph with two particles in it." That's when I said to myself, 'These people are crazy.'" (*SF* p.245) It's too bad that the NCI scientist didn't do more than just say truthful things to himself because these crazy people helped give us "Holocaust II."

Gallo still wouldn't back down in the spring of 1986 when, at an AIDS conference, according to Crewdson, he referred to "the Pasteur's contribution to the search for the cause of AIDS as inconsequential." (*SF* p.246) The Pasteur scientists gave as good as the got. One of their lawyers, Jim Swire, according to Crewdson, "upped the ante by accusing someone in Gallo's lab of having stolen LAV. 'They simply studied it,' Swire said, 'concluded we were correct, renamed it, and claimed it as their own.'" (*SF* p.247) Otherwise known as the classic Gallo Three-card Monte.

The person in Gallo's lab who would ultimately get hung out to dry for the handling of the fake discovery of HTLV-3, Mika Popovic, was eager to give investigators the impression that if anything untoward had happened, it was just an innocent mix-up. But according to Crewdson, the French were just not having any of that. (*SF* p.248) The bottom line for the French was that they wanted their "share of the patent royalties."(*SF* p.249) After all, Gallo had used *their* supposedly exogenous retrovirus to make his lousy test.

Things got even more sinister in this story when the lawyer for the Pasteur Institute used the Freedom of Information Act to try and obtain documents from Gallo's lab that would support the French case against Gallo's claims. According to Crewdson, "the memos that would have been most helpful to the Pasteur's case—and most detrimental to the government's—were withheld, in some cases without any indication that they even existed." (*SF* p.259) One of the withheld documents which Crewdson ultimately obtained, made it clear that Gallo had lied about *when* he had isolates of his so-called AIDS virus. (*SF* p.260) According to Crewdson, the most damning document that was withheld was a memo from Gallo about growing the French virus *at a time that he later insisted he had not been growing it.* (*SF* p.260) The only documents that seem to have been withheld were ones that supported the unavoidable conclusion, that Gallo was one of science's greatest pathological liars.

Joanne Belk, the government's person in charge of providing the documents requested under the Freedom of Information Act, described her interaction with Gallo to Crewdson: "I didn't know how rude he was . . . . This man called me and started blasting me on the phone. 'Who the hell do you think you are?' He was terribly profane. Nobody ever talked to me like that. That was my introduction to this so-called eminent scientist." (*SF* p.260) Gallo was totally uncooperative. Interestingly, in terms of the basic quality of Gallo's science, Belk's overall impression of his lab from a visit was that it was "impressively messy." (*SF* p.261) When Gallo finally did comply with the F.O.I.A. request, Belk got a call that she could pick them up at "Biotech Research laboratories in Rockville which Beck thought surpassingly odd." (*SF* p.262) One wonders, like so many other parts of this sometimes mysterious story, what was *that* about?

The documents that were turned over to Belk were very much in the Gallo lab's signature style. According to Crewdson, ". . . none of Popovic's pages was signed. Neither were any of the pages evidently kept by others in Gallo's lab.' (*SF* p.262) Most shockingly, considering his pivotal role in creating the scientific paradigm at the heart of "Holocaust II," "Popovic's notes, written in an unmistakable middle-European hand, resembled a diary or a journal, filled with retrospective observations and abbreviated descriptions of each day's work, but scarcely any experimental protocols or new data." (*SF* p.262) The lawyer for the Pasteur Institute is quoted by Crewdson as saying that the notes looked like they had been "shuffled like a deck of cards," and when he "tried to assemble the notes in chronological order, he found that the follow-up results for one experiment were dated three weeks before the experiment." (*SF* p.262) This was the orderliness of the abnormal, totalitarian, and sociopathic science of HIV/AIDS at its very best. According to Crewdson, one Popovic page "dated Jan 19, 1984 was continued on a page Nov 7, 1983." (*SF* p.262) The Mad Hatter would have been at home in a white coat at a workbench in Gallo's laboratory. Best of all, according to Crewdson, "Several of Popovic's pages weren't dated at all." (*SF* p.262) As was typical for a laboratory skilled at rewriting the past, Crewdson reports that several of the Popovic pages "were whited out" and "In a sequential log of laboratory specimens, the year '84' had been crossed out and replaced by '83.'" (*SF* p.262) That describes what they found, but according to Crewdson, once again the scarier thing was what the lawyers *did not find:* "In the notes that did exist, Swire and Weinberg could find no support for many of the experiments described in Popovic's *Science* article." (*SF* p.262) Swire could find no evidence of the isolation of the so-called virus from patients that Gallo had written about in his letter to *Nature* which was meant to exculpate him. (*SF* p.262) Most importantly, in terms of the French lawsuit, important documents reflecting the Gallo lab's work with the French retrovirus were missing, and one of Gallo's subordinates told Crewdson that the staff *had been told to leave them out.* Crewdson wrote, "to Swire, it looked as if somebody had systematically tried to replace the evidence of Popovic's work with LAV [the French virus] with something that would appear innocuous to the Pasteur's lawyers." (*SF* p.265) There was also evidence that the French virus had gone through a process of renaming in the documents *in order to obscure the origin of the virus the Gallo lab worked with.* (*SF* p.265) In many ways, disingenuous wordplay is at the heart of the deceptions of "Holocaust II."

None of this came as a surprise to Gallo's close observer and arch enemy in England, scientist Abraham Karpas, who watched all of this unfold in an "I told you so" mode. He told Crewdson, "Dr. Gallo still believes that in this age of communication and science he can get away with not only saying, but even writing, that black is white and vice versa." (*SF* p.269) If only people like Karpas, who seemed to astutely recognize that

Gallo lived psychologically in some kind of sociopathic opposite world, had gone a step or two further and realized that when Gallo often said that HIV was the indisputable cause of AIDS that "killed like a truck," he was also saying something akin to "black is white and vice versa." But that was a bridge too far.

As the noose tightened, Gallo went into advanced paranoia, suggesting that the lawyer for the French was "hiring people to come to restaurants to sit where I go to eat, to try and hear what I say." (*SF* p.271) Crewdson quotes one rant that makes Gallo sound like he had completely lost it: "I look at the French capitalizing on their food industry from some places where my ancestors came from . . . I think they do great in getting credit for nothing half the time, more than any people I've ever seen. That's the bias I would have against France . . . They helped us get into Vietnam." (*SF* p.273) Sound like anyone you know with weird hair?

One of the more revealing moments of Freudian projection in Crewdson's portrait occurs when he quotes Gallo telling the editors of *Nature* in an unpublished interview that Montagnier "hasn't a single collaborator left, because no one trusts him. I find him extremely political, always not sure what he believes. People who are full of distrust and see the world scheming to screw them. That's the way I look at the guy . . . Montagnier's an example of a small guy who stumbled into shit. And he got famous. More than he deserves. He can't handle it, sees everybody as plotting against him." (*SF* p.273) This from the most flamboyantly paranoid man in science, the man who was always accusing everyone of being out to get *him*. The real tragedy of "Holocaust II" was that the world was not and is not out to get *him*. At least not yet.

In the unpublished *Nature* interview, Gallo contradicted things that had been published in that very publication. According to Crewdson, "*Nature* had previously assured its readers that Gallo had grown LAV for one week only and in small quantity. Now Gallo admitted that LAV had grown for at least three months and there had been plenty of virus." (*SF* p.275) The fact that this vital information was never published is consistent with what we have said about the manner in which information is managed in the world of abnormal, totalitarian, and sociopathic science. Crewdson writes, "Had the Gallo interview been reported, it would have dramatically changed the face of the dispute with Pasteur. But *Nature* never published a word of what Gallo had said—or anything else about its investigation." (*SF* p.275) Gallo could even count on international protection for his sociopathic kind of science.

As the Gallo dispute with the Pasteur Institute got more cantankerous, the scientific community began to fear the collateral damage it was doing to the image of science itself. Legendary scientist Jonas Salk sought to lower the temperature of the conflict and according to Crewdson, he "spent the end of 1986 and the beginning of 1987 shuttling between Robert Gallo and Luc Montagnier in search of a shared version of history." (*SF* p.293) These scientists seem to have had a very abnormal idea of what history actually is. It is not the difference you split between two warring scientists, especially when one of the scientists is a world-class pathological liar. Eventually, according to Crewdson, "Jonas Salk had nearly given up hope of working out a history acceptable to both Gallo and Montagnier. 'Insanity afloat,' was the way Salk described the process to Don Francis." (*SF* p.295) "Insanity afloat," unbeknownst to Jonas Salk, was the best way to describe the all of the science and epidemiology of "Holocaust II." And it is still afloat.

Eventually, worn down, Montagnier stupidly agreed to a publication of a joint chronology of the discovery of the so-called AIDS virus with Gallo in *Nature*. As is typical of abnormal, totalitarian, and sociopathic science, it was published without any peer review which, according to Crewdson, "may explain why it contains a number of factual mistakes, why several names were misspelled and why portions of the text read as if they had been translated from Chinese." (*SF* p.296) And Crewdson notes that the chronology's preamble began with a real mutually-agreed-upon whopper: "Both sides wish it known that from the beginning there has been a spirit of scientific cooperation and a free exchange of ideas, biological materials and personnel between Dr. Gallo's and Dr. Montagnier's laboratories. The spirit has never ceased despite the legal problems and will be the basis of a renewed mutual cooperation in the future." (*SF* p.296) Beyond enjoying the hilarious absurdity of this big lie, one also starts wondering about the integrity of the French discoverers of the so-called AIDS virus. Note to future historians: Gallo apparently wasn't the only one willing to cut corners. The French may have also had something to hide.

Crewdson reports that despite whatever peace Gallo got from the pile of loopy revisionist lies published in *Nature*, he was soon disturbed by a new investigative piece in *New Scientist* written by Steve Conner. The article began, "In the war against AIDS scientific truth was among the first casualties. No one listened when Luc Montagnier at the Pasteur Institute in Paris said that he had found the virus that causes AIDS. Scientific journals and scientists preferred to hear what Gallo was saying from The National Cancer Institute in the U.S." (*SF* p.298) The article included Gallo's photos which had been misrepresented as HTLV-3 as well as the accusation that Gallo's outrageously dishonest behavior had cost many lives. Gallo's protectors didn't waste time coming to his rescue. Crewdson reported that one of Gallo's cronies, Dani Bolognesi, wrote a letter to his colleagues urging them to respond to the article. (*SF* p.299) And even the Reagan administration got involved in trying to get the French AIDS officials to join Health and Human Services in condemning the article, even though, as Crewdson points out, "no one could say what inaccuracies Connor's article contained." (*SF* p.299) Such awesome power can only make one wonder what Gallo had on the government that made the authorities so ready and willing to always come to his rescue. Was there a cat in the bag called "AIDS" that Gallo could always have let out? (See my book, *The Chronic Fatigue Syndrome Epidemic Cover-up*, if you want to hear that cat meow.)

When a settlement agreement was finally signed by the French—so that they could at least get their royalties for the AIDS test—they had to agree to renounce "any statements, press releases, charges, allegations or other published or unpublished utterances that overtly or by influence indicated any improper, illegal, unethical or other such conduct or practice by any scientists employed by HHS, NIH, or NCI." (*SF* p.299) The royalties the French would receive had officially become hush money. Crewdson notes, "With the stroke of a pen, the accusations and contentions of the past two years had been erased." (*SF* p.299) More importantly for the larger issue and the real history of "Holocaust II," the French *agreed not to tell the whole truth* about the history of AIDS, again making them in some ways not all that different from their American counterpart.

In the Gallo tradition of biting the hand that had saved him, Gallo, according to Crewdson, threatened the White House if they dared to try and take any credit for the mendacious agreement. (*SF* p.300) Who the hell did the American government think it was? After the bizarre, outrageously dishonest agreement with the French was signed, in a statement that should have made everyone who died of AIDS roll over in their graves, Gallo said, according to Crewdson, "Now, instead of being distracted by all the legal business, I'll be able to return full time to trying to do something about this disease." (*SF* p.301) In other words, the bad luck of the gay community (and the black community) was about to get much worse.

The agreement rankled the Pasteur team who felt that French politicians like President Chirac, who had put pressure on Pasteur to sign the agreement, had betrayed them. According to Crewdson, "Jean-Claude Chermann couldn't comprehend why someone who had chased the wrong virus for so many months was now being anointed in the press as the co-discoverer of the right virus." (*SF* p.302) Of course the whole situation was even wackier than Monsieur Chermann realized. His awesome date with destiny is still to come.

One of the absolute worst things that happened to the world as a result of the Gallo crime was that Gallo became the go-to spokesperson for AIDS science. According to Crewdson, "The settlement notwithstanding, the newspapers and magazines continued to laud Gallo as the discoverer of the AIDS virus while rarely mentioning Montagnier" and "whatever Gallo said was likely to make news." (*SF* p.310) He had become the Pope of AIDS under false pretenses. Even David Remnick, *The Washington Post* reporter who would years later become the ubiquitous editor of *The New Yorker*, had a warm shoulder for Gallo to whine on: Gallo complained to him that the settlement with the French had failed to end the "accusations" and "hatred" from some of his scientific colleagues. (*SF* p.310) In a hyper-ironic candid confession, Gallo said to Remnick, "I'm telling you, there are days when I wake up in the morning and feel like the Archangel Gabriel. By the time I go to bed at night, I feel like Lucifer. What's going on? Please tell me why they do this to me. Why do they say these terrible things about me? Do you know? Do you?" (*SF* p.310) Is it possible that deep down Gallo may have known himself that the questionable science of the HIV/AIDS paradigm was crafted in part by a Dr. Jekyll and Mr. Hyde?

Gallo's propensity for boilerplate homophobia kicked in a bit when Randy Shilts's book, *And the Band Played On* came out. Crewdson quotes Robert Gallo as saying, "It never ceases to me to be a source of great wonder . . . how people such as a gay young man on the West Coast think they know more when they're stimulated [sic] by the same two people over and over again. Namely Don Francis and what I would regard as a psychotic who lives in Cambridge." (*SF* p.311) In the heterosexist world of abnormal, totalitarian, "homodemiological" science that characterized AIDS, there was nothing more threatening than a "stimulated" gay reporter, especially one who had been "stimulated" by a psychotic. As for Gallo's ludicrous charge of psychosis clearly directed at his critic Abraham Karpas who was at Oxford, well, let's just say that science's largest glass house had rocks flying in every direction.

Gallo was so angry at the things that Randy Shilts quoted the CDC's Donald Francis saying about him that he penned a letter of retraction and he demanded Francis sign it. He told Francis that if he didn't (according to Crewdson), he had a "plan of action against Don Francis, which included evidence like letters and tape recordings, that would show financial impropriety in Francis's relationship with Randy Shilts." (*SF* p.313) One wonders: What, no gay sex? But wait. According to Crewdson, he also threatened to expose things from Don Francis's personal life. (SF p.313) Gallo was the J. Edgar Hoover of science with a real or imagined dossier on everyone. The long arms of this vindictive scientist are reflected in the fact that, according to Crewdson, "When it became clear Francis had no intention of signing Gallo's letter, word reached Berkeley [where he was happily working] that he was being transferred back to CDC headquarters in Atlanta—to work not on AIDS, but on tuberculosis." (*SF* p.313) It was the career equivalent of sleeping with the fishes.

Eventually, even Gallo's boss, Vince DeVita, tired of his antics. He told Crewdson, "there was always some crisis with Bob Gallo . . . He has an arrogance about him, that he felt he could talk to you and persuade you to his way of thinking. And he almost always failed." (*SF* p.314) Crewdson reports that Gallo, as per usual, refused to share his "AIDS" viruses and his cell lines which prompted people like Nobel Laureate David Baltimore to join another scientist, Howard Temin, "in worrying that Bob's way of handling himself does significant harm to both himself and to the national AIDS effort." (*SF* p.310) Baltimore and Temin were only aware of the tip of the iceberg. (Of course, Baltimore himself wasn't exactly the Mother Teresa of science.)

Gallo exhibited the censorious style typical of abnormal, totalitarian, and sociopathic science when a book which was critical of him by Michael Koch was published in Europe. Koch's book contained entertaining sentences about Gallo like, "He was so fond of his own ideas that he saw evidence where there was no evidence." (*SF* p.320) Koch in due course got the Gallo treatment. According to Crewdson, when Koch ran into Gallo at a scientific conference, Gallo told him, "Here is a five-step program to destroy you. You, your job, your position, your damned Carnegie Institute in Stockholm." (*SF* p.320) One thing you could say about Gallo is that even his rants had power points. (SF 320) One thing Gallo said about Koch underlines the danger of ceding absolute power to scientific elites. According to Crewdson, Gallo insisted, "I do not feel he was qualified to write such a book. Moreover, Koch has no experience in retrovirology . . ." (*SF* p.321) Perhaps the only person qualified to write about Robert Gallo was Myron Essex, Anthony Fauci, or Gallo himself. Or Professor Irwin Corey.

After Gallo's administrative assistant, Howard Streicher, wrote a threatening letter to Cambridge University Press, the firm that was going to publish the English language edition of the Koch book which had been first published in Germany, the book was cancelled. Streicher wrote in his letter that the book was "both maliciously damaging and likely to be scientifically, historically and medically unsound." (*SF* p.322) Translation: the book told the truth.

On the heels of the settlement with the French, a new Gallo scandal emerged. It turned out that the cell line Gallo's lab had supposedly created to grow the stolen French AIDS virus was also basically, well, stolen. Gallo had used his familiar modus operandi; he just changed the name of the cell line which had actually been created by a scientist named Adi Gardner and—Presto! Chango!—it was Gallo's. According to Crewdson, "When Gazdar told a Public Health Service lawyer he thought Gallo and Popovic had appropriated his discovery, he was advised not to pursue the matter. (*SF* p.333) Some scientists are said to have green thumbs because they are so good at growing things like viruses and creating cell lines. Gallo didn't need a green thumb. He had sticky fingers.

The idea that this character seriously thought he would win a Nobel Prize by operating in the manner he did challenges all definitions of sanity. Scientist Sam Waksal (who went to jail for the insider trading financial scandal that involved Martha Stewart) described a special night with Gallo in which "Gallo was drunk, and he had a tear in his eye, and he said, 'You know, I would do anything—anything—to win the Nobel Prize.' I always thought it was the most telling thing about him. Because in the world of science the goal is the pleasantry of the discovery and he could never find as much satisfaction in the discovery as he could in the limelight." (*SF* p.336)

There was still more public humiliation in store for Gallo when sophisticated genetic analysis of Gallo's so-called HTLV-3 made it painfully, embarrassingly clear that it was LAV and that whatever happened in terms of contamination or theft, *it had definitely all happened in Gallo's lab.* (*SF* p.341) And then the darkest moment of Gallo's travails happened on November 19, 1989 when John Crewdson's 55,000 word piece with all the details of his pseudo-discovery of the AIDS virus was published in *The Chicago Tribune.* The piece's conclusion was that "What happened in Robert Gallo's lab during the winter of 1983-84 is a mystery that may never be solved. But the evidence is compelling that it was either an accident or a theft." (*SF* p.343) Crewdson was being kind. Or the newspaper's lawyers were. *The Chicago Tribune* piece aired all of Gallo's dirty laundry, exposing him making bogus claim after bogus claim; it showed him perpetually rewriting history, and the article displayed his stealing-and-renaming habit as well as his penchant for deliberately altering scientific documents. As was typical of this master double-talker, according to Crewdson, in an interview about *The Chicago Tribune* piece, "Though [Gallo] claimed not to have read the *Tribune*, Gallo nonetheless took umbrage at a number of the quotes it contained." (*SF* p.344) What Crewdson had done in his amazing *Tribune* piece (and subsequently in his book) was to show the dark side of science: "The reality that scientists often engaged in the same kind of back stabbing and throat-cutting as politicians and businessmen had remained behind laboratory doors."(*SF* p.347)

As Congress began to slowly wake up to the general issue of fraud in science, the NIH had been guilt-tripped into creating "a new agency, the Office of Scientific Integrity" which was responsible for "investigating and deciding cases of suspected plagiarism, falsification, or other scientific misconduct." (*SF* p.349) In other words, all the dishes that could be found at the Gallo buffet table. After reading the Crewdson article on Gallo, the acting director of the new Office of Scientific Integrity decided that the Gallo affair deserved to be investigated." (*SF* p.351)

Even as the Gallo investigation was getting underway, he was out in the public serving up more scientific baloney. According to Crewdson, he "was at Fordham University in the Bronx where he announced a breakthrough discovery—a cure for Kaposi's sarcoma, the malignant lesions that account for about one in five deaths among AIDS patients." (*SF* p.354) The only problem, according to Crewdson, was that "Gallo hadn't published any such results, and he hadn't presented any data at Fordham to back up his claims." (*SF* p.354) In other words, for Gallo it was business as usual. When a desperate AIDS patient contacted one of the scientists in Gallo's lab he was treated badly. The man subsequently wrote a letter to the scientist and Crewdson quotes it: "You have probably forgotten our conversation . . . But I have not and I will not forget it in a long time. I have never in my life been talked to in such a demeaning, condescending, rude and abrupt manner by anyone let alone an alleged health care professional on the public payroll. I am dying from AIDS and in particular Kaposi's sarcoma . . . Which is what motivated me to call Dr. Gallo's office in the first place . . . How cruel it is to publicly talk about a cure and then refuse the information to the public." (*SF* p.354) Demeaning? Condescending? Rude? Cruel? When Gallo's boss heard about the exchange, he ordered Gallo to apologize to the man, and, according to Crewdson, "to explain that he didn't have a cure for Kaposi's sarcoma after all." (*SF* p.354) It was one of the few times that being Robert Gallo *didn't* mean never having to say you're sorry.

As the full-scale investigation of the Gallo affair by the Office of Science Integrity got under way, Gallo was fully cooperative. Not. Crewdson reports, "It had been early January of 1990 when Suzanne Hadley requested the originals of the Gallo lab's notebooks, but by mid-March she still didn't have them." (*SF* p.355)

Because of both Crewdson's *Tribune* piece and the OSI investigation, Monagnier felt emboldened to ignore the agreement to "ferme le bouche" and he admitted to *Le Monde* that there was a real possibility that Gallo had stolen LAV. (*SF* p.356) Gallo was furious and once again ran to the sympathetic *Washington Post* with his bogus version of the story. (*SF* p.357) (This was clearly *not* the same paper it had been during the Woodward and Bernstein era.) Gallo also hired a P.R. firm and a lawyer but, according to Crewdson, told his staff, "It should not be obvious that we are using a P.R. firm or a lawyer." (*SF* p.358) Abnormal, totalitarian, and sociopathic science cannot be conducted without a P.R. firm and a lawyer that agree to keep a low profile.

The list of property crimes committed by Gallo's gang expanded while he was under investigation by OSI when it was discovered that Zaki Salahuddin, the Gallo subordinate who was supposedly the co-discoverer of HBLV (eventually called HHV-6) had set up a company called PanData in order to funnel money into his own bank account by selling medical supplies to the National Cancer Institute—supplies which he himself ordered. (*SF* p.322) (At least he wasn't out stealing viruses, although, when the whole story of HHV-6 is told, that might not exactly be the case.) According to Crewdson, Congress got wind of the scam and John Dingell eventually called it "'a gross conflict of interest . . . on the part of a prominent AIDS researcher at the National Institutes of Health' who had hidden his 'improper financial interest in a biomedical firm doing substantial business with his own laboratory at NIH.'" (*SF* p.362) According to Crewdson, Gallo told the General Accounting Office that he knew about the Salahuddin company only three months before the investigation, but he told *The Washington Post* he had known about it for a year. (*SF* p.362) Crewdson reports that Salahuddin was also selling viruses and cell lines derived from Gallo's lab. One could say that abnormal science and abnormal commerce are bosom buddies.

Salahuddin was ultimately investigated by a Grand Jury. During his tribulations, Salahuddin said an all too true and disturbing thing about Gallo: "Here's Gallo, they provide him double coverage, internal investigation and so forth, all this moral turpitude he is accused for such a long period of time. No one ever talks of suspending him. In my case they go immediately for the knife and throw me to the wolves." (*SF* p.363) Salahuddin was eventually "formally accused of violating conflict-of-interest statues and accepting illegal gratuities in the PanData case." (*SF* p.375) As part of his punishment the was supposed to perform community service by researching HHV-6, the virus he purportedly discovered, which was a little like sentencing Bernie Madoff to selling stocks and bonds.

During the OSI investigation, more mind-blowing information surfaced. Mika Popovic provided a shocking description of his period in Gallo's lab: "When I came here nobody gave me whatsoever any instructions how we should write out notes or anything else. And when the litigation started, suddenly I was asked for notes." (*SF* p.364) That anyone in any way trusted the basic science that came out of this scientific pig pen is unbelievable. The OSI investigation identified new misrepresentations that Popovic had made in the *Science* papers that had supposedly nailed HIV down as the cause of AIDS. According to Crewdson, Popovic didn't have data to back up statements in the signature AIDS papers about patients he had described as showing evidence of reverse transcriptase. (*SF* p.364) (And the scientists who questioned the HIV theory were the really crazy ones. Go figure.)

According to Crewdson, in the course of the OSI investigation, Gallo's testimony basically revealed that he had misrepresented the truth during the period in which the government was aggressively and groundlessly defending him against the French lawsuit. (*SF* p.371) He admitted he had no AIDS virus before his lab got its hands on the French virus. (*SF* p.371) He also confessed he didn't have the isolates of the AIDS virus that he had bragged about at the time of his *Science* paper appeared. (*SF* p.371) It had all been just the usual Gallo malarkey. According to Crewdson, Gallo told the OSI that he had made the false claim about the isolates because "to be quite frank, I was nervous." (*SF* p.371) Crewdson points out that if Gallo had been as honest during the French lawsuit, Pasteur would have walked away with *complete ownership* of the patent of the so-called AIDS blood test. (*SF* p.372) And reporters might not have been calling up Gallo and hanging on to his every word of wisdom about AIDS.

A panel drawn from the Academy of Science that was called in to oversee the OSI investigation voted to move the OSI investigation from an inquiry to "a formal misconduct investigation of Gallo and Mika Popovic." (*SF* p.373) They were shocked by "the apparent lack of supporting data for Popovic's key experiments." (*SF* p.373) The Academy of Science panel didn't realize that they were conducting an investigation in the opposite world of abnormal, totalitarian, and sociopathic science. One of the panelists noted—about the basic work on the AIDS virus done in Gallo's lab—that "It may not be that you will be able to find a written record of all the data that are in print." (*SF* p.374) One could say that the data that helped build the HIV/AIDS paradigm of "Holocaust II" wasn't worth the paper it was *not* written on.

Gallo kicked and screamed when OSI went so far as to requisition materials that had been used in the original AIDS experiments. When Suzanne Hadley arrived to collect those materials, according to Crewdson, she "felt like the vampire surrounded by angry villagers." (*SF* p.375) She told Crewdson, "His whole lab, they just worship Gallo and will not challenge him. Anybody who gets a bunch of people around him who gets a mindset that he can do no wrong and that everybody else is wrong and wants to get him, you know that's a prescription for disaster. Because nobody is asking the tough questions on the inside." (*SF* p.375) Gallo's own description of his gang in Crewdson's book is quite revealing: "About seventy-five percent of the people with me are from foreign countries, their salaries are twenty to thirty thousand dollars, they're M.D.-Ph.D.s, they work day and night, they work seven days a week." (*SF* p.385) It would appear that the virological fraud that helped create "Holocaust II" may have been crafted in what could be deemed a scientific sweatshop. What Zaki Salahuddin said about Gallo's rosy prospects during the investigation deserves close scrutiny by anyone trying to understand the nature of Gallo's political power: "Nothing will come out of it. No one wants America to go down. They just rally around the flag. NIH and Gallo are inseparable right now. If he goes down, NIH goes down." (*SF* p.376)

One of the more amusing moments in the Crewdson book concerns an NPR radio show on which *Business Week* reporter and author Bruce Nussbaum was being interviewed during the promotion for his book on AIDS, which according to Crewdson, purported "to show that Wall Street and NIH had conspired to slow the approval of potential AIDS drugs." (*SF* p.384) One of the people calling into the radio show attacked Gallo by name, saying that he had "'done a disservice to research in general.'" (*SF* p.384) Gallo just happened to be listening to the radio and he angrily called the show. When Gallo started going on and on about how he and his associates had risked their lives doing AIDS research and basically suggested that Nussbaum didn't have "a depth of understanding of science," (*SF* p.385) Nussbaum responded, "I think you're expressing the type of attitude which is part of the problem. . . . You simply dismiss anyone who is criticizing NIH in any way." (*SF* p.385) He also said, "Your attitude is one of incredible arrogance . . . . I think you're really expressing the type of attitude that is really at the core of the problem of the NIH. And you're not open to criticism . . . . Even if that criticism is valid. You simply dismiss all criticism as invalid." (*SF* p.386)

Popovic's defense of himself during the OSI investigation continued to provide evidence that Gallo's lab had the rigorous organization of a town dump. According to Crewdson, he told investigators that he had been "working under a great deal of pressure, under very difficult conditions, and without technical support," and he complained that the equipment was of "poor quality." (*SF* p.387) Unfortunately, we now know that the science that came out of that equipment was of the same quality. He complained that the seminal AIDS virus articles in *Science* had been written in his bad English very quickly because of intense pressure from Gallo. (*SF* p.387) And the world would live with the tragic effects of that bad English and that rush job for many decades.

The Office of Scientific Integrity wasn't buying anything Popovic was selling. The committee was especially concerned about a key falsehood in the original *Science* papers which was that the French virus LAV hadn't been growing in the Gallo lab at the time the so-called Gallo virus, HTLV-3, had been discovered. Popovic betrayed the boss by saying that *he* wasn't the one who wrote the offending sentence in the *Science* paper and according to Crewdson, that basically left Gallo as the chief suspect. (*SF* p.389) Popovic had dared to be honest about the matter. He is quoted by Crewdson as telling OSI, "I am sure that originally I had referenced the LAV in my very rough draft. Even I think I insisted on it. I thought that we should include the LAV data in the paper . . . . Then it was changed in the editing . . . LAV was put to the end of the manuscript, in the end, and I think it was Dr. Gallo's decision not to include LAV." (*SF* p.389)

While this investigation was underway, another scandal broke out in the Gallo lab. Gallo's deputy lab chief, Prem Sarin, had taken money under false pretenses from a company that wanted Gallo's lab to test a potential AIDS drug called AL-721. (*SF* p.390) Sarin, according to Crewdson, was convicted "of embezzlement and making false statements to the NIH" and he "got two months in a halfway house in Baltimore." (*SF* p.391) While he had been under investigation, his fellow financial felon in the Gallo lab, Zaki Salahuddin, had urged Sarin to avoid going to jail by spilling some beans on Gallo, but given Gallo's psychological and professional iron grip on his staff *that* would never happen. (*SF* p.391) It will fall to future historians to determine the nature of the beans that were never spilled and what bearing they might have on the true and complete narrative of the AIDS era.

Peter Stockton, an aide to Congressman John Dingell, was amazed to see Gallo get off while his subordinate was nailed. (*SF* p.399) When Dingell's committee staff interviewed Gallo about his responsibility for all the financial misbehavior in his lab, Stockton, according to Crewdson, said that Gallo excused himself by saying, "'Hey, come on, it's not my job to be doing that kind of thing. I'm a scientist and I'm trying to cure AIDS, and I can't be bothered with this kind of crap.'" (*SF* p.392) And Stockton's committee basically said back to Gallo, according to Crewdson, "Somebody's got to be concerned about this. You just don't turn laboratories over to felons to run wild. You've got to keep some control over what's going on." (*SF* p.392) What Stockton didn't realize was that AIDS research in general had been turned "over to felons to run wild." Gallo was an iconic role model for everyone in that field. He was their Fagin.

The Pasteur Institute eventually published a paper in *Science* that settled the matter genetically and established conclusively that LAV and Gallo's supposed discovery were the same virus and that everything Gallo had said about the matter was a crock. It was the beginning of the end of Gallo at N.C.I. He had embarrassed the whole NIH. (*SF* p.402-403) But with Gallo there was always time for one more scandal and the next one may have been his ugliest one yet because it involved the deaths of human guinea pigs. Gallo had gotten involved with French researcher named Daniel Zagury in a research project that involved testing experimental vaccines on Africans. And not just any Africans—the test subjects were children. In the course on testing the vaccine, there were three deaths. Gallo and "Zagury had failed to mention that in the report on the vaccine." (*SF* p.406)

One of the most fascinating revelations in Crewdson's book is the fact that while using LAV in his experiments, Popovic was so afraid that Gallo might screw the French that he had given his sister in Czechoslovakia "the early drafts of the *Science* article for safe keeping" because, according to Popovic, "I believed that sometimes in the future I might need them as evidence to prove that I gave fair credit to Dr. Montagnier's group." (*SF* p.411) According to Crewdson, "the hidden manuscripts suggest that Gallo was guilty for his rewriting of Popovic's paper." (*SF* p.411) Popovic clearly knew all too well what Gallo was capable of.

The OSI report which was drafted by Suzanne Hadley stated that both Gallo and Popovic were guilty of scientific misconduct. (*SF* p.414) But when the higher ups saw it, they balked and *wanted the guilty verdict against Gallo erased.* (*SF* p.414) Gallo once again ducked the bullet. But Gallo didn't go completely unscathed. According to Crewdson, the OSI report "said that Gallo's behavior 'had fallen well short of the conduct required by a responsible senior scientist and laboratory chief.' Gallo had 'acquiesced in Dr. Popovic's wrong doing.' He 'may even have tacitly encouraged, and at a minimum, he did not discourage, the conditions that fostered the misconduct.'" (*SF* p.418) What was actually fostered in those conditions was far worse than anyone could have imagined.

Suzanne Hadley, according to Crewdson, felt that the conclusions of OSI supported the perception that Gallo had lied under oath during the dispute with the French over the AIDS virus patent. (*SF* p.419) She was upset when her superior, NIH Director Bernadine Healy, wanted her to rewrite her report. (*SF* p.420) She asked Healy to make the request for a change in writing and warned that it would compromise "the OSI independence from NIH." (*SF* p.420) Healy then backed down. But Hadley would pay a price for standing up to her boss. She was told she was being "reined in" and would make no more "decisions in the Gallo case." (*SF* p.421) Crewdson notes that previous to her involvement with the Gallo case, Hadley "had been one of the NIH's rising stars." (*SF* p.420) But given her perception of Healy's power and temperament, Hadley completely withdrew from OSI's Gallo case, saying, according to Crewdson, "The hell with it, I just want to get rid of it. I don't need this shit anymore. . . . I never wanted anything out of this . . . except to do it right. But I certainly never wanted to get just absolutely destroyed. I would have been demolished by Bernadine. She absolutely would have destroyed me." (*SF* p.422) That's what happens in abnormal, totalitarian, and sociopathic science in general when one tries to tell the truth or do the right thing.

When the OSI report was released, Gallo got the kind of cover he often received from an uncritical press. According to Crewdson, "The Associated Press declared Gallo's vindication," and said nothing about the Popovic misconduct verdict. (*SF* p.422) Crewdson reports that all that Healy did to Gallo was issue a directive ordering him to "'familiarize himself with all

HHS and NIH regulations relevant to his job, including standards of conduct for federal employees and the rules governing medical experiments on human subjects.'"(*SF* p.423) Gallo was also, according to Crewdson, ordered "to review 'all primary data' produced by any scientist under his supervision before the data was submitted for publication, and to ensure that his assistants maintained 'written laboratory notebooks and records sufficient to permit scientific peers and supervisors to adequately interpret and duplicate the work.'" (*SF* p.424) If such rules had been in place for Gallo—and followed—*before* he got his mitts on AIDS research, HIV may never have become the central fraud of "Holocaust II."

Gallo decided to set the record "straight" in his inimitable style by writing a book called *Virus Hunting*, which was as flattering to himself as one would expect, and according to Crewdson, was a project in which he didn't even get Montagnier's first name correct. (*SF* p.429) According to Crewdson, "Buttressed by scant documentation, Gallo's book was drawn mainly from his own recollections and those of his staff. Perhaps for that reason, it frequently left the impression that some insight or discovery occurred sooner than it did." (*SF* p.429) It was interesting that according to Crewdson's account at least one member of the French team seemed to also be capable of playing the kind of games that Gallo played. Crewdson writes that "a preface by Jean-Claude Chermann recounting the discovery of LAV . . . read as though Chermann had done it single-handedly." (*SF* p.430) One begins to wonder if any leading scientist during the AIDS era got enough love and attention as a child.

According to Crewdson, when the OSI report came out, the "publicity in Paris" inspired the Pasteur Institute to consider "the possibility that the 1987 agreement [with Gallo] would have to be renegotiated." (*SF* p.430)

Looking back on her work on the Gallo OSI investigation, Suzanne Hadley, according to Crewdson, was most "dismayed" by her failure "to get an early handle on the full compass of the case—to see how some of the entries in Mika Popovic's notes, or some of the phrases in his *Science* article, while seemingly disconnected might have implications in a larger context for the patent, the blood test, the veracity of the Reagan administration, and the settlement with the French." (*SF* p.434) Crewdson reports that she said, "It was so much bigger than we imagined. Once I began to get my wits together, it was too late." (*SF* p.434) Crewdson summed up the dilemma: "So broad was the scope of the Gallo case that it seemed ludicrous in retrospect, to have attempted to fit it into the narrow framework of a scientific investigation, which typically focused on the misreporting of an experiment in a published article. Even more than whatever had happened in Gallo's lab, Hadley was appalled by the government's behavior, in and out of court." (*SF* p.434) Hadley told Crewdson, "Whatever one thinks about Gallo . . . he had support all the way up the line. They had data back in 1984 showing they were the same virus . . . There never was an iota of a chance that HHS would do an honest thing. Before anything had even happened, the die was cast, the decision was made. After that it was simply a matter of crafting a litigation strategy." (*SF* p.434) Hadley deserves great honor for doing the right thing but even her intense epiphany about Gallo and the outrageous fraud she was staring at was just scratching the surface. Beneath the mendacities by Gallo and the Reagan administration concerning *who* discovered the so-called AIDS retrovirus lay far more catastrophic secrets and lies that would ultimately blossom into a world of HHV-6-related immune dysfunction.

When the scientific community saw the watered down OSI report— which Crewdson described as almost completely changed from the Suzanne Hadley version (*SF* p.436)—with its main misconduct charge focused on Popovic, and Gallo once again ducking the main bullet—many were horrified. But *The Washington Post*, once again played the role of Gallo enabler and declared Gallo vindicated. (*SF* p.436) One scientist, Gene Myers, when he heard Gallo was still not willing to admit that his discovery was actually the French retrovirus, is quoted by Crewdson as comparing Gallo to Dostoyevsky's Karamazov. (*SF* p.436)

When Bernadine Healy met with the panel that was overseeing the final watered-down OSI report, one of the members described what she said to them and it was chilling and ironic. Crewdson quotes Alfred Gillman's account of Healy's remarks: "What she wanted to know . . . is does Gallo have no redeeming qualities at all? Is this guy the scum of the earth? Or is there a spark of genius there that ought to be nourished? Or is he mentally ill?" (*SF* p.438) One can reasonably guess that the victims of "Holocaust II," voting from their graves, would probably vote "no" on redeeming qualities, "yes" on scum of the earth, "not so much" on spark of genius and "absolutely yes" on mentally ill.

While *The Washington Post* bent over backwards to help Gallo, ABC's Sam Donaldson went in the other direction when he took up the story. Donaldson's TV report began, "It may be the greatest scientific fraud of the twentieth century." He also warned that "important elements of the United States government seem reluctant to have all the facts revealed." (*SF* p.442) If he only knew. Donaldson was just one more reporter who didn't see the even more important issue lurking beneath the surface of the LAV story.

One of the most disturbing moments in the government's peculiar protection of Gallo, and one that should be pondered and investigated by historians of "Holocaust II" for many decades to come happened when Congressman John Dingell's office began their investigation of the Gallo affair. Dingell brought the beleaguered Suzanne Hadley into his congressional investigation of Gallo because she knew where all the Gallo bodies were buried. But when the committee requested the files from the preceding OSI investigation she herself had conducted, it turned out that notebooks from the investigation *had been shredded by Hadley's replacement at OSI.* (*SF* p.461) Gallo was a cat with more than nine lives. Abnormal and totalitarian science had abnormal and totalitarian oversight.

For anyone who believes that some kind of bizarre group psychosis characterized the whole enterprise of AIDS research, it is of interest that when Peter Stockton talked to famous Nobel Prize winning scientist James Watson during this period about Gallo, according to his account in Crewdson's book, Watson's "big point was that Gallo is a manic depressive. He thinks the subcommittee should back down because Gallo's crazy. He thinks we should talk to Gallo's shrink." (*SF* p.473) One could say that to comprehend all the pseudoscientific underpinnings of AIDS or "Holocaust II" one must talk to Gallo's shrink.

As could be expected in the arbitrary and opposite world of AIDS science, OSI itself was changed into the Office of Research Integrity and the rules were changed even while the Gallo investigation was ongoing—just like the rules of science were altered by bogus AIDS research. Instead of simply finding scientists guilty of publishing fabricated scientific results, under the new rules the committee had to show that the scientists who was charged *had intended to do so.* (*SF* p.466-475) That ridiculous new standard made it nearly impossible to find any scientist guilty because, according to Crewdson, the scientist "could simply claim he hadn't intended to deceive anybody." (*SF* p.454) Gallo's most powerful Guardian Angel had arrived on the scene in the form of this crazy new rule. Another dark legacy of AIDS and "Holocaust II" would be that the government's process of trying to defend Gallo would make it easier for *all* American scientists to commit fraud and get away with it. Gallo was truly an historic figure in that he paved the way for many more years of plausibly deniable scientific fraud. It is a breathtaking legacy.

Even with the rules of evidence loosened in Gallo's favor, he continued to behave like a cornered Mafioso as he told scientists who were expected to testify before the new committee that if they testified it might not turn out too well for them. (*SF* p.499) He told one scientists that he might "spill the beans on him." (*SF* p.480) Gallo was a virtual Boston of spillable beans.

The final OSI report on the Gallo affair was basically a whitewash, a true-blue cover-up. Suzanne Hadley described it as a "version of history" that "parroted the government's arguments years before in defense of the blood-test patent." (*SF* p.503) She told Crewdson, "There's too much pseudoscience in the opinion. They got it from somewhere." (*SF* p.503) Again, what Hadley didn't grasp was how catastrophically deep the pseudoscience laid out before her was.

When an appeals board reversed the verdict of the ORI, Gallo was elated. According to Crewdson, Gallo said, "I will now be able to redouble efforts in the fight against AIDS and cancers. There are several hopeful new avenues of AIDS research that my laboratory is pursuing." (*SF* p.505) The business of "Holocaust II" could continue in earnest. *The New York Times* reporter, Nicholas Wade, one of the AIDS paradigm's truest believers, wrote that Gallo was "the one scientific hero who has yet emerged in the fight against AIDS." (*SF* p.505) With heroes like that, gays, blacks and anyone suffering on the HHV-6 spectrum illnesses didn't need enemies.

But John Dingell wasn't done with Gallo. His staff attempted to get prosecutors to charge Gallo and Popovic with making false statements under oath, but between complications involving the statute of limitations for the crime and problems of involving the jurisdiction the crimes took place in, that never happened. (*SF* p.510) Bullet ducked again.

All of this mishegas took its toll on Gallo's new boss, Sam Broder, who had succeeded Vincent DeVita. According to Crewdson, "Since replacing Vince DeVita, Sam Broder had defended and protected Gallo. Now there were indications Broder, like DeVita before him, was growing disillusioned. Reportedly, horrified by Daniel Zagury's use of Zairian children in his AIDS vaccine research, Broder had ordered Gallo's name removed from the pending HHS patent on Zagury's vaccine. When Suzanne Hadley showed Broder Gallo's outrageous statement that the patent had been initiated by Broder himself, Broder exploded, He said, 'That's bullshit!' Hadley recalled." As if that wasn't enough, according to Crewdson, Hadley used the same meeting with Broder to tell him that her investigation "had turned up evidence that several of Gallo's subsequent articles also contained false statements." (*SF* p.514) Hadley told Broder about a paper Gallo published in 1985 which contained false statements about the AIDS virus isolates he had in 1982. According to Crewdson, "The paper was a political exercise, a pollution of the scientific literature intended to help lay the groundwork for a defense against the French." (*SF* p.515) Crewdson reports that Sam Broder told Gallo that if he didn't retire he would order a new NCI investigation of him. (*SF* p.515) Suzanne Hadley is quoted by Crewdson as remembering that Broder said to her, "I told Bob, 'You've degraded the institute, you've degraded the public and you've degraded reporters by lying to them. . . .We owe things to the people of another time. They need to know what things were really like during the era of AIDS research.' One of Bob's biggest sins is his overdriven compulsion to claim all the credit and to trace it all to his great intellect." (*SF* p.515) As true as Broder's words were, he was still missing the sin beneath the sin, not the sin of stealing credit, but the sin of egotistically leading the world down a deadly misbegotten path, manipulating science and the public into thinking he had delivered the truth about AIDS to the world. And as far as *that* sin was concerned, Broder himself was joined at the hip with Gallo.

As quoted by Crewdson, something else Hadley remembered Broder saying sizzles with irony: "He was confused out of his mind. Bob was so thoroughly wrong. The AIDS virus had to fit the retroviruses as he knew them, and he was wrong. He needed to listen to his data, and he did not want to do that . . . Bob writes all these historical things that have no relationship to the way it really was. I told Bob, 'I have not forgiven you for this. People are dying of real diseases, and this is not a game.' . . . Frankly Suzanne, it was a Nobel Prize run. You guys don't talk about that, but I was there, and I know. And frankly he almost got it. And if he had gotten it, he would have been truly invincible." (*SF* p.516) Where to begin? Well, first of all, Gallo's word of choice for the people this science involved, at least on occasion (as reported by *New York Native*), was "fag" which may have had a little something to do with the level of moral seriousness with which Gallo dealt with the AIDS issue. Second of all, who is Broder to talk? He was the scientific genius behind the aggressive pushing of AZT into the bodies of AIDS patients, something akin to pouring gasoline on a fire.

In 1994 there was a revised settlement with the French which Crewdson described as "a clear victory for the French." (*SF* p.585) Suzanne Hadley, working for the Dingell Committee, wrote a 267-page account of the whole matter that according to Crewdson "spared no one" in assigning culpability "starting with the Department of Health and Human Services." (*SF* p.526) Crewdson writes that the report said that "HHS did its best to cover up the wrongdoing" and "meanwhile the failure of the entire scientific establishment to take any meaningful action left the disposition of scientific truth to bureaucrats and lawyers, with neither the expertise nor the will essential to the task. Because of the continuing HHS cover-up it was not until the Subcommittee investigation that the true facts were known, and the breadth and depth of the cover-up was revealed. . . . One of the most remarkable and regrettable aspects of the institutional response to the defense of *Gallo et. al.* is how readily public service and science apparently were subverted into defending the indefensible." (*SF* p.527) As profound and disturbing as the report was, it was naively focused on only the tail of a far bigger unseen monster, namely the "HIV-is-the-cause-of-AIDS" mistake itself and the entrenched world of abnormal, totalitarian, and sociopathic science that it represented. The report was clueless about the psychotic and deeply biased paradigm at the very center of "Holocaust II." It was commendable for Dingell, Hadley, and Stockton to nail Gallo on the viral theft from the French, but relatively speaking, it was in essence a successful prosecution of a misdemeanor that missed the exponentially more important underlying medical and scientific crime against mankind.

To say that Gallo landed on his feet after this disgrace is an understatement. When he left NCI he had to rough it at the brand new, built-just-for-him, multi-million dollar research Institute of Human Virology in Baltimore financed by the state of Maryland. And as one could expect in the opposite world of Robert Gallo, one of the people he invited to come work for him at the spiffy new institute was the paragon of great science, Mika Popovic, a man who will probably take some of Gallo's juiciest secrets to the grave with him. Gallo's ability to either discover things or steal them, depending upon how you looked at his career, seems to have diminished in Baltimore. According to Crewdson, "During its first five years of life the Institute for Human Virology hadn't come up with any marketable discoveries." (*SF* p.537) AIDS patients were clearly safer with Gallo out of NCI and eating crab cakes in Baltimore.

Near the end of his account of the Gallo affair, Crewdson writes his most chilling sentence: "The Popovic-Gallo Science paper, among the most-cited scientific articles of all time, is laden with untruths that have never been retracted or corrected." (*SF* p.539) In other words, the very foundation of "Holocaust II" is laden with untruths that "have never been retracted or corrected." Every living scientist and doctor should hang their head in shame. They are the apathetic, compliant "ordinary Germans" of this period in history. And anyone who describes *Science* as a prestigious publication worthy of any kind of reverence at all should put on a pair of clown shoes.

Crewdson closes his awesome dissection of Gallo's misdeeds and character on a philosophical note: "Being wrong in science is hardly a sin. Scientists are wrong every day, and their mistakes are what pushes science forward. What set Gallo apart, was his profound disinclination to acknowledge his mistakes, preferring instead to ignore them, insist they hadn't occurred, blame someone else, or propagate outlandish explanations and outright fictions that only confused science further and slowed its forward march . . . . In the end, the most compelling question was one only Gallo could answer: Had he somehow convinced himself that all the lies were true? Or had he known better all along?" (*SF* p.540) Actually, a more fundamental and philosophical questions would be whether Gallo was capable of honestly answering that question or even understanding it. Was Gallo a true sociopath? And that leads to the larger historical question about the degree to which a kind of enabling group psychosis and sociopathology went way beyond Gallo and underwrote all of "Holocaust II." It may have taken a whole psychotic village to empower a Gallo.

While the world owes journalistic genius John Crewdson a debt of gratitude for laying bare the mind-numbing complexities of Gallo's scientific fraud regarding the discovery of the so-called AIDS virus, the larger story that Crewdson missed, the one he failed to see beneath all the masks that he successfully did rip off, was the game-changing story that the so-called stolen AIDS virus *wasn't even the cause of AIDS*. While Crewdson was writing his masterpiece, which was ultimately published in 2002, evidence was accumulating that the other virus that Gallo claimed to have discovered, HHV-6, actually *did play a major role in AIDS*. In fact, *the* major role. The virus was not an unimportant pathogen as portrayed by Crewdson in *Science Fictions*.

The *New York Native*, the little gay newspaper that pioneered the Gallo story even before Crewdson got to it, followed the HHV-6 trail that led to a far bigger and more disturbing story about AIDS than just Gallo's appropriation of LAV. While covering HHV-6, the *New York Native* broke one of the biggest AIDS stories of all, the breakout of acquired immune deficiency in the general population which the CDC and the NIH hid behind the ridiculous euphemism of "chronic fatigue syndrome." The *New York Native*'s reporter, Neenyah Ostrom covered chronic fatigue syndrome, AIDS and their relationship to HHV-6 from 1988 until the paper went out of business at the beginning of 1997.

The parent company of *New York Native* published three books on Ostrom's reporting about the relationship between HHV-6, AIDS and chronic fatigue syndrome. The first book, *What Really Killed Gilda Radner? Frontline Reports on the Chronic Fatigue Syndrome Epidemic*, was published in 1991. In the book's introduction, Ostrom wrote "For whatever reasons— like reluctance to admit the presence of another AIDS-like epidemic sweeping the nation in the shadow of (and linked to) the official AIDS epidemic, simple incompetence, or more sinister reasons—health authorities have tried to deny the very existence of the chronic fatigue syndrome epidemic in the U.S., have tried to prove that the illness of immune dysfunction is caused by 'psychoneurosis,' [and] have delayed for years determining how many cases actually exist in the country . . . ." (*WRKGR* p. 10) The next Ostrom book, *50 Things You Should Know About the Chronic Fatigue Syndrome Epidemic* was published in 1992. In its introduction, she wrote, "America is facing a health crisis of unprecedented proportions, a crisis that has been misleadingly labeled chronic fatigue syndrome. This health crisis has been bungled by government health officials from the very beginning: It has been ignored, misrepresented, and investigated ineptly until, as I write this in January, 1992, untold millions of Americans already have contracted this potentially disabling, AIDS-like illness. . . . CFS is clearly an AIDS-related illness that puts the entire population at risk." (p.13-14) The final Ostrom book, *America's Biggest Cover-up*, which was published in 1994, was even more uncompromising in its conclusions. Ostrom attempted to explain why officials refused to admit a link between AIDS and chronic fatigue syndrome: "AIDS patients, and people who test HIV-positive (whatever that actually turns out to mean), have been so badly treated, so discriminated against, so scapegoated and demonized that it is not surprising that there is an almost reflexive recoiling from the possibility that AIDS is not the narrowly-defined illness that it has been portrayed as being." (*ABC* xvi) She asserted that "Until the denial among medical professionals about the relationship between the AIDS and chronic fatigue syndrome epidemics is overcome, however, it is difficult to imagine how either epidemic can be ended." (*ABC* xvi) Had John Crewdson not just taken the lead on Gallos's theft of HIV from *New York Native*, but also followed the trail of Ostrom's reporting on chronic fatigue syndrome and HHV-6, he might have broken a bigger and far more important story.

Two years before Crewdson's book on Gallo hit the bookstores, Nicholas Regush's book on HHV-6, *The Virus Within: A Coming Epidemic* was published. Regush had been a reporter for the *Montreal Gazette* as well as an award-winning and Emmy-nominated medical and science journalist at ABC News, where he produced segments for World News Tonight with

Peter Jennings. Regush's book covers the history of HHV-6 from its discovery through a succession of shocking discoveries made by two researchers at the University of Wisconsin, Konnie Knox and Donald Carrigan. Regush's picture of HHV-6 bears little resemblance to the failed Gallo co-factor of Crewdson's book.

The HHV-6 story that emerges from Regush's book should have made the scientific community's collective head spin. In a series of experiments on a variety of patients, the two relatively young Wisconsin researchers showed, without even fully admitting it or shouting it out to the world, that *HHV-6 was the real villain in AIDS*. They showed that HHV-6 is capable of wreaking havoc in both the central nervous system (*TVW* p.9) and the immune system itself. Prior research by R.G. Downing had shown that HHV-6 was capable of destroying T-cells (curiously, the only so-called herpes virus to do so) which was something that the AIDS establishment insisted on blaming HIV alone for doing indirectly even though HHV-6 destroyed the cells dramatically, directly and unambiguously. As Regush pointed out, "Here was a herpes virus that could destroy T-4 lymphocytes at least in the test tube more powerfully than HIV." (*TVW* p.54) Had Crewdson dug deeper on the HHV-6 story, he would have learned that there are supposedly two strains of HHV-6, an A and a B strain. And he would have found out that HHV-6A was indeed starting to look more and more like the significant co-factor in AIDS or even more surprisingly, like *the chief viral culprit itself*. Gallo wasn't lying about the power of HHV-6. According to Regush, "In November 1993, Robert Gallo's lab published data gleaned from autopsies of five people who had died of AIDS, demonstrating an abundance of HHV-6 infection. Footprints of the virus were found in areas such as the cerebral cortex, brain stem, cerebellum, spinal cord, tonsils, lymph nodes, spleen, bone marrow, salivary glands, esophagus, bronchial tree, lung, skeletal muscle, myocardium, aorta, liver, kidney, adrenal glands, pancreas and thyroid." (*TVW* p.84) If anything, Gallo was underestimating the power of HHV-6 in order to keep his beloved stolen virus HIV alive. Ironically, one of the reasons Gallo didn't do more work on HHV-6 during the 80s was because he was busy fending off investigations from Congress and journalists like Crewdson (and pesky newspapers like *New York Native*.)

One of the early HHV-6 research projects conducted by the Wisconsin researchers showed that HHV-6 is a major lung pathogen in AIDS, a fact that tragically had been largely ignored in the treatment of AIDS. And one of the most important findings on HHV-6 that could have an impact on everyone's health was Carrigan and Knox's determination that "Direct infection of the [bone] marrow by HHV-6" was possible (*TVW* p.62) According to Regush, their research showed "that HHV-6 could infect— and suppress—bone-marrow cells." (*TVW* p.64)

While Konnie Knox was focusing on HHV-6's relationship to HIV, her research actually began the shocking process of pulling the rug out from under HIV itself. Her work with Carrigan showed that HHV-6 could also seriously dysregulate monocytes and macrophages, making it a very creative and dangerous *AIDSish* pathogen. (*TVW* p.68) She made HHV-6 the subject of her doctoral thesis and Regush reports that she wondered if she was "throwing herself into the hurly burly of Big Science politics." (*TVW* p.69) Actually, she was throwing herself into the hurly burly of Big Abnormal, Totalitarian, and Sociopathic Science politics.

Knox started sealing the deal for HHV-6's role in AIDS when she studied tissue samples of a group of people who had died of AIDS. According to Regush, "The results of her experiments gave her a jolt: all 34 tissue samples of lung, lymph node, liver kidney and spleen revealed that at the time of death there was active HHV-6 infection as opposed to merely a biological sign that the virus was 'latent' (embedded in tissue)." (*TVW* p.83) Her experiment also showed that one of the big AIDS showstoppers, CMV, wasn't even as important because she found it active in only nine of the 34 tissue samples. (*TVW* p.84) Most alarmingly in terms of the way lung issues had been treated in AIDS was the fact that she found evidence in some of the patients that HHV-6 was probably responsible for the destruction of the lungs. (*TVW* p.84)

Knox, not knowing the real nature of AIDS politics, told Regush that she was "amazed that so little HHV-6 research had actually been done on AIDS patients . . . . It didn't make much sense." (*TVW* p.85) She was another scientist who had found her way into HIV/AIDS Wonderland. She didn't have the right compass for the science of opposite world or the nasty retroviral and heterosexist (and racist) politics that had laid its foundation.

The profile of HHV-6 as a virus capable of destroying the immune system was dramatically increased when, according to Regush, "various labs exposed HHV-6 as" capable of targeting T-8 cells and when scientists at the National Cancer Institute showed that "HHV-6 infects and kills natural-killer cells. These are the immune cells that destroy abnormal cells in the body, particularly those that are infected by viruses. HHV-6 is the first virus known to be capable of targeting and seriously damaging such a vital element of the immune system's antiviral defenses." (*TVW* p. 87) (The fact

HHV-6 was capable of killing natural-killer cells should have alerted the whole scientific community to the link between AIDS and chronic fatigue syndrome which are both low natural-killer cell syndromes. It should have also raised the question of whether HHV-6 should be in a different viral category. It increasingly seemed *sui generis*.)

Knox found that HHV-6 "could cause major damage during the early development of AIDS," (*TVW* p.89) *and didn't need HIV to do it*. According to Regush, "Her autopsy-tissue study had already shown that macrophages were often depleted in the lungs of HIV-infected AIDS patients," and she was determined "to know how HHV-6 was capable of knocking out those cells . . . . Her tests showed that, besides destroying macrophages, HHV-6 interfered with the normal functioning of the scavenger cells by blocking the release of a type of oxidant, a substance that cells normally generate to attack microbes. Knox noted that HIV was not known to be capable of this specific type of action." (*TVW* p.95) She concluded that HHV-6 had the potential to destroy the macrophages in the lungs *without HIV*, a totally sacrilegious idea in the abnormal science of AIDS. According to Regush, she dared to wonder heretically if HIV was "doing any killing in the body, or was HHV-6 the lone assassin?" (*TVW* p.96)

Knox also found that HHV-6 was capable of causing brain infection or encephalitis without any signs that HIV was involved. (*TVW* p.97) And the same no-show behavior on the part of HIV occurred in the case of the bone marrow in AIDS: "Knox's lab studies demonstrated that HHV-6-infected marrow cells—not the HIV infected ones—blocked the ability of the marrow to produce mature, differentiated cells." (*TVW* p.97) The same scenario was manifest when she looked at the brain damage in AIDS patients. Regush writes, "When Knox studied the brains of six people who died of AIDS and found extensive damage in four to their nerve fiber sheaths she also detected active HHV-6 infection. The infected cells were only in areas where the damage had occurred and never unhealthy tissue. The damaged tissue tested negative for signs of HIV, CMV, and other microbes. Again, there was only HHV-6." (*TVW* p.101) According to Regush, all of this inspired the very dangerous doubt in Carrigan and Knox about whether "HIV was even necessary for AIDS to occur." (*TVW* p.101)

The pièce de résistance of the Knox and Carrigan research involved the lymph nodes of AIDS patients. According to Regush, "the development of AIDS has largely been viewed as a progressive destruction of the networks of lymphocytes and fibers known as the lymphoid tissue. AIDS scientists, however, have been unable to associate the presence of HIV in the lymph nodes with any damage to the tissue." (*TVW* p.98) While the conventional wisdom was that HIV was hiding in the lymph nodes and destroying them, what Knox and Carrigan found turned the conventional wisdom upside down. In perhaps their most important study they found that "16 lymph-node biopsies from HIV-positive patients all contained cells actively infected with HHV-6A. Twelve of 16 patients who had been diagnosed with progressive disease had more dense infection that the four patients who had been diagnosed as having a stable condition. Knox and Carrigan also found more dense infection in areas where the lymph nodes were losing lymphocytes than in areas free of destructive change or where normal tissue in the nodes was already being replaced by the formation of scar tissue. HHV-6 was the apparent cause of the destruction of lymphoid tissue that occurred in these HIV positive people." (*TVW* p.114) Regush didn't mince words about the implications: "HHV-6 was not only at the scene of the crime, but it appears to have committed the crime as well." (*TVW* p.114) Regush describes Knox and Carrigan as wondering if they had found a "smoking gun" because "there were no convincing studies demonstrating that HIV could cause similar pathology." (*TVW* p.114) They submitted their research to *The Lancet*, but as could be expected, it was not accepted. It was ever thus during "Holocaust II."

In the world of Kuhnian normal science Carrigan and Knox would have had their Nobel Prizes by now for showing that HHV-6 was the real AIDS virus and was even more important than just that as other research began to connect it to many other diseases that would turn out to be part of an HHV-6 spectrum of disorders. But not in the opposite world of abnormal, totalitarian, and sociopathic science that was dominated by the heterosexist and racist HIV/AIDS paradigm. HHV-6 threatened the whole epidemiological house of cards the CDC and the NIH had presented to the world. Good luck to future HHV-6 scientists and historians all over the world when they try to put Humpty Dumpty back together again.

In an interview with Robert Gallo, Regush asked him about Knox and Carrigan. Regush reported, "Gallo spoke very generously about what Knox and Carrigan had accomplished, but he also emphasized that they work in too much obscurity to obtain any funding. 'They have clearly shown that HHV-6 is a powerful pathogen,' Gallo said. 'If they were headliners at a major university, it would make a huge difference.'" (*TVW* p.223) How two scientists who were essentially doing a controlled demolition on the HIV/AIDS paradigm could ever even hope to be allowed positions of prominence in a scientific world dominated by disingenuous scoundrels like

Gallo requires a huge stretch of the imagination. As Regush concluded, their research "suggests that HIV may not always be necessary as a companion to HHV-6 when the herpes virus is destroying tissue. But even suggesting that in writing would raise the hackles of HIV researchers. In fact, some AIDS scientists compare any questioning of the HIV hypothesis as it currently stands, to denial of the Holocaust. With such emotions running strong in AIDS science, why take a chance of boldly presenting alternative hypotheses?" (*TVW* p.224) Unfortunately for the world, Regush reported that Knox and Carrigan didn't have the stomach to go more public with their story or to join forces with the AIDS critics and dissidents: "Knox and Carrigan, while aware of the issues, want no active part of this often hostile debate." (*TVW* p.224)

It was very unfortunate that the brilliant, tireless John Crewdson never found his way into this shocking HHV-6 part of the AIDS story. His exposé of Gallo and the purloined retrovirus had caught the eye of the NIH's investigative body and Congress itself. Had Crewdson found his way to the Knox and Carrigan laboratory at the University of Wisconsin and done the same kind of Pit Bull due diligence on the primary role of HHV-6 in AIDS, he might have helped bring "Holocaust II" to an early end and everything would have been different for people on the HHV-6 spectrum. And knowing how Gallo had stolen HIV, Crewdson might have eventually looked into the allegations that he also stole credit for discovering HHV-6, which is another story. And just as creepy.

The Four Doctors of the Chronic Fatigue Syndrome Apocalypse

How the Bigotry and Incompetence of Four Scientists at the Centers for Disease Control Helped Create the Chronic Fatigue Syndrome Disaster

Introduction

During the last several decades, I have known four remarkable women with a serious illness that has been given the extremely deceptive diagnostic label of "Chronic Fatigue Syndrome." Three of the women are still "living" with the illness. "Living" with Chronic Fatigue Syndrome generally means facing a cascade of disturbing medical events that leave them in a constant state of dread about what will happen next. One of the women was so incapacitated that she had to travel around on a motorized scooter and she was killed when she was hit by a truck on her way back from the grocery store. Chronic Fatigue Syndrome is such a hellish disease that there are those with the illness who would sardonically say that she is one of the lucky ones. All four of the women had very promising futures ahead of them. They outclass me in so many ways that they probably would not even give me the time of the day had they not been stricken with Chronic Fatigue Syndrome and met me because of my interest in the subject.

I was the publisher of a newspaper that is credited with doing the first major reporting on the AIDS epidemic. My newspaper, *New York Native*, was a relatively new gay publication in New York City when I got a phone call about a strange pneumonia affecting gay men in New York City. I asked a doctor to investigate and he wrote a story in which the New York City health authorities said that the rumors were unfounded. Several weeks later, that all changed when a *New York Times* story appeared in which the CDC confirmed that indeed, a strange illness seemed to have broken out in the gay community. I detail my newspaper's coverage of the emerging epidemic in my book *The Chronic Fatigue Syndrome Epidemic Cover-up*.

The early reporting in my newspaper is almost universally praised. In *Rolling Stone*, David Black said that the paper deserved a Pulitzer prize. Also in *Rolling Stone*, Katie Leishman wrote, "It is undeniable that many major stories were Ortleb's months and sometimes years before mainstream journalists took them up." In his bestseller, *And the Band Played On*, Randy Shilts wrote, "Because of the extraordinary reporting of the *New York Native*, the city's gay community had been exposed to far more information about AIDS than San Francisco in 1981and 1982."

But the love affair with *New York Native* quickly fizzled out as my newspaper dug deeper into the story. Our early reporting was fairly straightforward and, in retrospect, typical of most medical and scientific reporting then and now. It basically translated semi-arcane information provided by government and establishment officials for a lay public. It was not particularly skeptical. As time went on, our reporting became more investigative and we began to notice serious problems with the competence and honesty of scientists at the Centers for Disease Control and the National Institutes of Health. It didn't help when I learned that one of the top AIDS researchers referred to gays as "faggots." When I learned that particular scientist and his close colleague at Harvard were both considered to be crooks by serious scientists in Europe, all bets were off.

One of the transformative moments for me and *New York Native* occurred when one of my readers sent me a clipping of a curious article in the March 25, 1986 issue of the *Los Angeles Examiner* by Ben Stein. *In Truth to Power*, I reported, "Stein wrote that it seemed to him that everyone in Los Angeles seemed to be sick at the time. People would develop a flu which lasted two weeks and then they would recover. But then a few weeks later they would get sick again. He described 'a vague, spaced-out feeling, chronic fatigue just over your shoulder, always breathing down on you, a susceptibility to wild upsets of the bowels all became part of daily life.' Stein complained that even though an incurable flu seemed to be spreading throughout Los Angeles, no one was doing anything about it. Public health officials were silent. Stein also wrote, 'Already my friends in the East tell me the non-stop flu has hit Washington and New York in a big way. This nation can be genuinely disabled by these incurable diseases. The individuals who have them are severely pained, physically and psychically. Having the flu half your life hurts, take it from me. Can anyone help? Isn't this worthy of national attention? Are we just going to have the stock market go up forever while everyone gets incurable viruses? I'm scared.'"

That mysterious flu, of course, turned out to be Chronic Fatigue Syndrome. It gradually became clear as day to me that this was the part of the AIDS epidemic that the Centers for Disease Control did not want the general public to know about because it would suggest that the CDC did not know what it was doing and the real epidemic could cause mass panic. (It has become evident over the last four decades that controlling panic is part of what most top public health officials would describe as a major part of their job description.) The idea that Chronic Fatigue Syndrome was another face of the AIDS epidemic became solidified when Hillary Johnson penned a two-part series on what would turn out to be Chronic Fatigue Syndrome in *Rolling Stone* in the summer of 1987. I had a total sense of "Eureka" when I read her articles and didn't rest until I tracked her down and shared idea that AIDS and Chronic Fatigue Syndrome were Tweedledum and Tweedledee, linked together not by HIV, but rather by a virus called HHV-6 which had the misfortune of being discovered in AIDS and Chronic Fatigue Syndrome patients after the book had been closed on the HIV theory of AIDS.

One of the most controversial series of stories that my newspaper broke involved our coverage of a distinguished scientist, Peter Duesberg, who raised serious questions about the HIV theory of AIDS. I ran stories about Duesberg numerous times on the cover of *New York Native*. You could say that Duesberg was the kid who said the Emperor had no clothes on, but this kid had a "genius grant" from the National Institutes of Health and was considered to be doing Nobel caliber work. As I watched Duesberg's critique suffer the slings and arrows of the powerful and corrupt scientific establishment, I began to fully understand how political science is in general, and how sinister the politics of AIDS are in particular. While I don't agree with everything Duesberg has to say about AIDS, I try to give his critique of HIV the respect it deserves in my book, *The Duesbergians*. And the political attacks on Duesberg are part of the inspiration for my book *Iatrogenocide: Notes for a Political Philosophy of Science and Epidemiology*.

The more my newspaper covered the connection between AIDS and Chronic Fatigue Syndrome and the HHV-6 challenge to the HIV theory of AIDS, the more controversial it became. One Nobel Laureate let me know what the scientific community thought of *New York Native* when he said to me on the phone, "If it's in your newspaper I know it's not true." And it wasn't just the AIDS medical and scientific establishment that wanted us to shut up. The AIDS activist group, Act Up, which posed as a revolutionary group demanding more funding for AIDS research, turned out to be just a de facto street mob arm of the AIDS establishment. Their supposed activism and angry performance art were essentially premised on the government's AIDS paradigm. I got a taste of what they were really up to when Peter Duesberg was about to share his ideas about with a Presidential committee in the 80s and Act Up members stood up to boo him. They were not only out to silence Duesberg. Eventually they voted to boycott my newspaper and they played no small role in the eventual demise of *New York Native*. I refer to the AIDS activists as "the Blackshirts" in my play about the AIDS epidemic, *The Black Party*.

I always held out hope that my newspaper would receive support from the Chronic Fatigue Syndrome community. We made a mark on journalistic history by assigning a writer, Neenyah Ostrom, to cover Chronic Fatigue Syndrome in virtually every issue of my paper starting in 1988. Article after article showed the connections between Chronic Fatigue Syndrome and AIDS. We also published three books by Ostrom, *What Really Killed Gilda Radner?*, *50 Things You Should Know about the Chronic Fatigue Syndrome Epidemic*, and *America's Biggest Cover-up*. While we were doing that, the Centers for Disease Control and the so-called AIDS Czar, Anthony Fauci, the Director of the National Institutes of Allergy and Infection Diseases, were refusing to even admit that CFS was a real medical condition, let alone another face of AIDS. With a few notable exceptions, the Chronic Fatigue Syndrome community was not happy about our reporting on the links between AIDS and Chronic Fatigue Syndrome.

In a way, the fact that AIDS has never ceased to be a "gay disease" in the public mind is confirmed by the resistance of the Chronic Fatigue Syndrome community to even discuss the obvious AIDS and CFS connections. I've said on numerous occasions that members of the CFS community would rather die that admit they are in anyway linked to the AIDS epidemic. And, unfortunately, more than a few have. I think I have learned more about the degree to which heterosexism and homophobia are hardwired into our science and culture from the CFS community than I have from any other stories about homophobia that my gay newspaper covered in its fifteen years of publication.

In some ways, because my gay newspaper paper did the world's most extensive coverage of HHV-6, you could say that it became an honorary "gay virus" in the minds of many members of the CFS community. Even if it was destroying every cell in their body (and it clearly was multisystemic) many wanted no part of it. When an intellectual and CFS activist reported that her Ampligen (a CFS drug) treatments seemed to make her better when they were controlling her HHV-6 infection, she was basically ignored by the community. I should point out that many in the community have also evolved into believers that they are not carriers of a contagious *anything*, so that also prevents HHV-6 from being taken seriously. A contagious "gay virus" associated with gay AIDS? OMG! Better to come up with theories of spontaneous CFS combustion than that!

While the CFS community refuses to deal with the evidence-based connection between CFS and AIDS and the reality of highly pathogenic HHV-6 in their beleaguered bodies, a virtual clown car of opportunistic scientists has arrived on the scene. Every few months it seems like some new scientist announces that *he or she alone* is taking CFS seriously and all the previous work is strictly amateur hour. An adult has finally entered the room! The newbie scientist then focuses on some small part of what is clearly a multisystemic disease and seduces the patients into thinking that he or she is on the path to "the truth." One prominent geneticist who entered the field tried to raise awareness about Chronic Fatigue Syndrome by wearing his underwear outside of his clothes. And after two eminent scientists at Columbia University, Mady Hornig and Ian Lipkin, made a dramatic entrance into the field, they helped garner more attention for CFS when according to *The New York Post*, Dr. Hornig alleged that Dr. Lipkin "repeatedly dropped his drawers and demanded she diagnose a lesion on his butt" and "kicked her under the table at meetings to keep her from speaking; presented her work as his own, and kept her from getting tenure."

And, of course, every colorful new Pied Piper leads the patients further and further away from the AIDS and CFS connection and the role of HHV-6, "the gay virus." A kind of medical AIDS/CFS apartheid is maintained that is a fool's paradise full of CFS corpses. And while everyone is not looking, the HHV-6 epidemic gets bigger and bigger and manifests itself in new ways. Just look at autism. (But that is another long story.)

One of the big problems for the CFS issue is that a big streak of authoritarianism runs through the community. There is a great deal of abject bowing and scraping to the government's medical authorities. The constant cry for more research money begs the question of the legitimacy of the recipients of all the research gold. I've often said that CFS needs less money and *more* honesty and forthrightness. The CFS community does not realize that they are victims of a major cover-up which is a biomedical *crime involving deceit*. This is a job for whistleblowers, not hapless activists who think at worse this is a crime of neglect that only requires more money and attention.

And so, we continue to find ourselves in very dark times that are perilous for truth and truthtellers. The real nature of the HHV-6, AIDS, and Chronic Fatigue Syndrome catastrophe is an inconvenient truth. We are now in the third generation of people who are affected by HHV-6. I have written this book in hopes that some members of the new generation will not be blinded by the prejudices that have prevented their parents and grandparents from seeing what is before their very eyes. If scientific clarity and moral courage can't be found, a new generation of HHV-6 and CFS victims will be condemned to a perpetual wild goose chase in a biomedical Tower of Babel.

This little book is a work of reverse-engineering. It takes the reader back to the beginning of the AIDS epidemic to show all the formative parts of the infernal machine that Chronic Fatigue Syndrome patients are trapped in. It all begins with a handful of scientists at the CDC whose incompetence and prejudices built the unmovable AIDS paradigm that now threatens everyone's health. My reverse-engineering of this mess shows that the inexorable Chronic Fatigue Syndrome train wreck originates in the misjudgments involved in the nosology, epidemiology and virology of AIDS.

And it didn't have to happen. In Hillary Johnson's masterful book about Chronic Fatigue Syndrome, *Osler's Web*, there is a discussion of an Atlanta doctor I actually think I may have talked to back in the 80s. In 1984, Richard Dubois reported in a medical journal on cases of what turned out to be Chronic Fatigue Syndrome. According to Johnson, "DuBois had first observed the phenomenon in 1980." (*Osler's Web*, p. 6) An important year for anyone who knows the history of the AIDS epidemic. And he didn't keep it a secret from the Centers for Disease Control. Johnson notes, "Richard DuBois had made a presentation to agency staff on the malady early in 1983, even proposing that the new mono-like syndrome might be a second epidemic of immune dysfunction rising concurrently with AIDS." (*Osler Web*, p. 31)

"Concurrently" is what this writer calls whistling in the dark. Why didn't anyone at the CDC (which is also in Atlanta) consider the real possibility that this other AIDS-like epidemic wasn't just "concurrent" but was yet another presentation of AIDS? Hopefully, by the time the reader finishes this book, the "why" will be painfully obvious.

*

A few definitions and elaborations are in order.

I coined the term "homodemiology" to describe epidemiology that is inherently homophobic and heterosexist. It is epidemiology that is always poised to blame epidemics on gay people. This book does not deal with the racist aspects of the AIDS paradigm. I use the term "Afrodemiology" for that. I have tried to capture the racism of AIDS in my novella, *The Closing Argument*.

To describe the nature of AIDS science, I use the words, abnormal, totalitarian, and sociopathic interchangeably. I use abnormal to capture the dark side of what Thomas Kuhn refers to as "normal" science. Kuhn has played a major role in my thinking about science and it is my little homage to him. "Sociopathic science" is fraudulent, conscienceless science. I explain my concept of "sociopathic science" more fully in my book, *Iatrogenocide: Notes for a Political Philosophy of Science and Epidemiology.*

I often refer to the AIDS epidemic as Holocaust II. While gays were not the primary target in "The Holocaust," they have that dubious honor in Holocaust II.

For more background on HHV-6 go to my site, HHV-6 University.

For more information on the *New York Native* visit New York Native University.

Randy Shilts and the Keystone Kops of AIDS

"Human destiny involves no greater misfortune than for the most powerful men on earth to be less than first-rate. Then everything becomes false, distorted and monstrous.

—Nietzsche

"And it is much easier for the aristocrat to be ruthless if he imagines that the serf is different from himself in blood and bone."

—George Orwell

". . . society has discovered discrimination as the great social weapon by which one may kill even without bloodshed.

—Hannah Arendt

At the center of the unfortunate mythology of the early part of the AIDS epidemic stands Randy Shilts, the gay reporter from the *San Francisco Chronicle* and the author of a highly successful book that some people, mistakenly, think is the definitive history of the early history of "AIDS." *And the Band Played On*, was for many years considered the rock solid account of the first four years of the "AIDS" epidemic. Wikipedia summarizes Shilts's biography: "Shilts graduated near the top of his class in 1975, but as an openly gay man, he struggled to find full-time employment in what he characterized as the homophobic environment of newspapers and television stations at that time. After several years of freelance journalism, he was finally hired as a national correspondent by the San Francisco Chronicle in 1981, becoming 'the first openly gay reporter with a gay "beat" in the American mainstream press.' Coincidentally, AIDS, the disease that would take his life, first came to nationwide attention that same year, and soon Shilts devoted himself to covering the unfolding story of the disease and its medical, social, and political ramifications." *And the Band Played On* is described in Wikipedia: as "a best-selling work of nonfiction written by San Francisco Chronicle journalist Randy Shilts published in 1987. It chronicles the discovery and spread of HIV and AIDS with a special emphasis on government indifference and political infighting to what was initially perceived as a gay disease that has impacted the United States and the world for decades after."

Insofar as the history of the science and politics associated with the first years of the epidemic were filtered through the journalistic judgment of Randy Shilts, one could say that epidemiological folly was compounded by journalistic folly. But to be absolutely fair, one can not underestimate the importance and usefulness of the basic raw facts reported in Shilts's book, even if they are naively framed and misunderstood by their author. Amid the wooden-headed (and unintentionally hilarious) credulousness of Shilts's conclusions throughout *And the Band Played On*, are reliable historical bits and pieces necessary for future historians who try and reconstruct an accurate myth-busting history of the epidemic and Holocaust II. A corrective forest needs to be put together from Shilts's credible trees.

When "AIDS" came to the medical community's attention in 1981, it was as though a small car called the Centers for Disease Control pulled up to the curb of the American public's consciousness and a gaggle of heterosexist clowns emerged who would craft the government's response to the epidemic and inadvertently lay the groundwork for Holocaust II, the HHV-6 catastrophe and the devastating age of autism. Randy Shilts's book is an important guide to *who* those biased clowns were and what they were thinking or perhaps more importantly, *what they were not thinking.*

Donald Francis: Scientist Zero

In many ways, Donald Francis, the epidemiological superstar of Shilts's book is also the star of the titanic HIV mistake that led to the HHV-6 spectrum catastrophe. Shilts's unfortunate hero worship begins with this description of the man: "Although he was only thirty-eight, Dr. Don Francis was one of the most eminent experts on epidemics at the CDC, having been among the handful of epidemiologists who literally wiped smallpox off the face of the earth in the 1970s." (*ATBPO* p.73) Harvard retrovirologist Myron Essex thought Francis "had gained an international reputation for singular brilliance." (*ATBPO* p.73) The colorful crew that crafted the official AIDS paradigm in the early 80s was off to a great start as a rather grandiose mutual admiration society. That might have been an early telltale sign of a groupthink catastrophe in the making.

Donald Francis had worked with Essex at Harvard on feline leukemia. No more precise nucleus of the tragic HIV mistake can be found than the moment when Francis (according to Shilts) *decided* that Gay Related Immunodeficiency (GRID, as it was known early on) was feline leukemia in people because both diseases were marked by weakened immune systems and opportunistic infections. Feline leukemia is *not the only animal disease to behave that way*, but Francis's myopic familiarity with feline leukemia would tragically keep all other more likely possibilities at bay while he pursued his pet theory under the guidance of his Harvard mentor and future Harvard AIDS millionaire.

A sure recipe for hubristic mischief could be found in the fact that Francis seemed so *very* sure of himself and his intuitions. He was also very sure that other people with their competing ideas for the aetiology of the mysterious epidemic were dead wrong. According to Shilts, "Francis didn't think the gay health problems were being caused by cytomegalovirus or the other familiar viruses under discussion. They had been around for years and hadn't killed anybody. It was something new; it could even be a retrovirus, Francis said." (*ATBPO* p.73) Saying it "could be a retrovirus" was disingenuous because other possible causes that were not retroviral were not welcome at the table. Ironically and tragically, Shilts foolishly celebrates this determined rush to judgment: "Francis was already convinced. He quickly became the leading CDC proponent of the notion that a new virus that could be spread sexually was causing immune deficiencies in gay men." (*ATBPO* p.74) Both epidemiology and virology were rather quickly being carved into stone with horrific consequences. One can now see the seeds of the Chronic Fatigue Syndrome epidemic and the HHV-6 pandemic in this misjudgment.

Donald Francis was the human embodiment of a stern, uncompromising public health message that can be heard constantly playing over the P.A. system throughout *And the Band Played On*. The questionable behavior of all other scientists at the time and what Shilts perceives as the self-destructive dithering of gay leaders is judged harshly against what Shilts considers the courageous, take-no-prisoners approach of Francis during epidemics he had previously worked on: "Years of stamping out epidemics in the Third World had also instructed Francis on how to stop a new disease. You find the source of contagion, surround it, and make sure it doesn't spread." (*ATBPO* p.107) Couldn't be any simpler than that. But nobody, Shilts included, was stopping to ask if Francis was fighting the last epidemiological war rather than the new one.

The Don Francis no-nonsense approach, a manly approach, was one Shilts clearly admires. While Francis will be the voice of moral testosterone throughout *Band*, according to Shilts's black and white schema, it falls to the gay community to play the role of denial-ridden, weak-kneed, self-destructive imbeciles. In the dark days of the early epidemic only the wise-beyond-his-years Francis *sees the light* and knows what to do. The Francis buzz word is "control." Dr. Donald Francis knew how to "control" epidemics. If only the dopes at the top of the nation's AIDS effort (and the epidemics uncooperative gay victims) had let him take control.

Francis's African experiences were epidemiologically formative. He had worked on Ebola Fever in Africa in 1976 and he will now look at this new disease through Ebola-colored glasses: " . . . the disease [Ebola] was a bloodborne virus, wickedly spreading both through sexual intercourse, because infected lymphocytes were in victims' semen, and through the sharing of needles in local bush hospitals." (*ATBPO* p.118) Shilts also looks at "AIDS" and public health itself through Francis's Ebola glasses: "When it became obvious that the disease was spreading through autopsies and ritual contact with corpses during the funerary process, Dr. Don Francis, on loan to the World Health Organization from the CDC, had simply banned local rituals and unceremoniously buried the corpses. Infected survivors were removed from the community and quarantined until it was clear that they could no longer spread the fever. Within weeks, the disease disappeared as mysteriously as it had come. The tribespeople were furious that their millennia-old rituals had been forbidden by these arrogant young doctors from other continents. The wounded anger twisted their faces." (*ATBPO* p.118) This passage is a key to understanding the moral of *And the Band Played On*, and the theme Shilts also promulgated in his publicity campaign for his bestselling book. It becomes the schtick he will hector his own community with. For "tribespeople" fill in the word "gays." If only the government had acted, had done something, anything, sooner. But what? Clearly Shilts wanted the country, under Dr. Francis—as a kind of extra-political AIDS Czar—to go into the same emergency mode reflected in the kind of ritual-banning measures he took toward the benighted tribespeople in Africa. In a manner of speaking, in a perfect Donald Francis public health universe, gay rituals (i.e. sex) would be banned, infected people would be removed from the community and quarantined. Whenever anyone will talk about the government not doing enough after *Band*, what will always be disingenuously unsaid is *what a heavy-handed government could have done if it had wanted to*. In the name of doing something—anything—involving a not much loved minority, things could have gotten extremely dicey in the inconvenient Bill of Rights sense, and there is nothing about what one detects in the character of either Francis or Shilts in the book to suggest that they would have done anything other than cheer such a development on. Gay men performed many foolish, politically self-defeating acts throughout the epidemic, but applauding Shilt's silly message about the heterosexist government of a heterosexist country *not doing enough*, with all its dark unconsidered implications of what draconian things might have been done in the name of dealing with a public health emergency, is surely one of the most foolish. Anything done under the biased auspices of Don Francis during the early days of the epidemic, can now be appreciated as an example of an incompetent government with questionable motives *doing too much too fast and using poor judgment*.

The impatient Dr. Francis considered the ideas of those at the National Institutes of Health who were looking at alternative theories like amyl nitrite or sperm as the cause of AIDS to be "ludicrous." (*ATBPO* p.119) Instead of suffering these fools, Francis set up his own laboratories and went to work to lay down the foundation for what would turn out to be the CDC's greatest epidemiological and virological mistake in its history. As for gay people, like the indigenous people of Francis's African epidemics, "Customs and rituals would have to be dramatically changed, and he knew from his hepatitis work in the gay community that customs involving sex were the most implacable behaviors to try to alter." (*ATBPO* p.119) Yeah, changing gay customs is like herding LGBT cats.

Shilts portrays Francis as a man of destiny: "Don Francis viewed his life as an accumulation of chance decision that had put him in the right place at the right time." (*ATBPO* p. 128) In retrospect, perhaps destiny had brought together exactly the wrong man, the wrong institution, the wrong epidemic at the wrong time to create the most perfect coalescence of misbegotten epidemiology and virology in history. Shilts swoons over the synchronicities of the Donald Francis life journey thus far: "By chance after chance, Don Francis felt he had been delivered to this moment in early March 1982, when it all fit together. The retrovirology, the cat leukemia, the experience with African epidemics, and the long work with the gay community—it all let him see something very clearly." (*ATBPO* p.128) Oy vey.

Francis looked through the world through the cockamamie *retroviral* lenses of Myron Essex. Francis had completed his doctorate on retroviruses and he was like the hammer that sees the world in terms of nails. It is a curious factoid of history that originally Francis thought that AIDS was co-factorial: Shilts reports he said, "Combine these two diseases—feline leukemia and hepatitis—and you have the immune deficiency." (*ATBPO* p.129) If Francis had only kept his co-factorial notion alive, there would have at least been a small chance that the HIV mistake might have corrected itself quickly rather than rolling out thirty years of hell on earth. Co-factors might have kept the great minds of epidemiology from closing.

To Francis, the conclusions were painfully obvious, and it was also clear what needed to be done. The Center for Disease Control needed "to launch some educational campaigns among gays to prevent the disease." (*ATBPO* p.129) The Great White Doctor had arrived among the ignorant, indigenous gays of America. The gay "implacable" behaviors had to change. Cut to the gay versions of "twisted faces" and "wounded anger" Shilts described in Africa. The CDC's age of epidemiological brainwashing had begun.

Often when a detective makes a major wrong turn, the suspect is right there in front of him. In Francis's attempts to fulfill the destiny of his retroviral dissertation, he overlooked the most obvious viral suspect of all, the one the size of a barn that was just staring at the CDC researchers, begging to be discovered. Francis memorialized this Missed Opportunity when he himself wrote in one of the very first books on the epidemic (a collection of essays on AIDS edited by Kevin Cahill), "Blood sampling of the intravenous drug users also revealed that although many were infected with cytomegalovirus, the viral strains were different. This was strong evidence that this herpes virus, which many scientists considered a strong candidate for a causative agent, had not developed some new virulent strain." (*The AIDS Epidemic, Edited by Kevin Cahill, St. Martins Press, 1983 p.*) No single strain emerged, lending further weight to Don Francis's hypothesis that a new virus, not CMV was at work. If only he had wondered if there was some new *DNA virus* that resembled CMV in some way that was hidden in the mix, the retroviral obsession might not have ultimately ruled the day. We know now that they were staring at HHV-6 and not seeing it. It would have been recognized as a new virus and probably declared the leading suspect. And then of course the HHV-6 spectrum pandemic and Holocaust II might never have happened. But it did.

Anyone who disagreed with Francis during this early period of the epidemic was considered stupid or stubborn. (This is how eras of abnormal and totalitarian science get their start in putative democracies.) We're constantly told throughout Shilts's book that Francis hoped "somebody would see how catastrophic the epidemic *would* become." (*ATBPO* p.147) Ironic, when you consider that indeed an apocalyptic catastrophe was coming and Francis himself was inadvertently taking a leadership role in making the key mistakes that would help to make it happen.

An amusing note is struck when Shilts points out that Francis wanted more labs to work on "AIDS" research because "they might get off on a bum lead and retard research at a time when people were dying." (*ATBPO* p.151) Francis, as it turns out, might live to see his name become synonymous with bum leads, and as far as dying is concerned, the show had only just begun.

There is no place that Shiltsian worship of Francis wouldn't go. He even followed Francis to bed: "The dream came to Don Francis often during those long, frustrating nights in the gathering darkness of 1982. Just beyond his reach, a faint orange light was suspended, shimmering with promise. It was The Answer, the solution to the puzzle. He reached for it, stretching so he could draw the light toward him. But it drifted farther and farther out. The answer was always there before him, tantalizingly close, and still beyond his grasp. Don's wife usually awoke him at that point. His mournful groaning would disturb the kids." (*ATBPO* p.159) Or, perhaps, in retrospect, it was just indigestion.

Our dreamer-scientist is portrayed as the solitary man of reason in an obstinate, irrational world: "The logical science of GRID (gay-related immunodeficiency) demanded that logical steps be taken . . . or people would die needlessly. However, as would be the case with just about every policy aspect of the epidemic, logic would not be the prevailing modus operandi." (*ATBPO* p.170) "The logical science of GRID" is perhaps the most oxymoronic phrase in the history of phrases. In what sounds now like ironic chutzpah, Shilts had the nerve to write, "Science was not working at its best, accepting new information with an unbiased eye and beginning appropriate investigations." (*ATBPO* p.171) From a Kuhnian promontory, one must ask, *whose* unbiased eye it is, *who* decides what is appropriate? But why even bother accepting new or contradictory information if you're being beamed up to "the Answer" by an orange light?

By January 1983, Don Francis is pounding his fists on tables. He is enraged at the blood banks. No one was doing enough to "control" the disease. There were fools full of denial everywhere and people shortsighted enough to express concerns about trifles like civil liberties in the face of the mounting death toll. Shilts, as usual, opined that the "problem, of course, was that such considerations constantly overshadowed concerns of medicine and public health." (*ATBPO* p.224) Public health logic is inexorable and very useful for those in the emotional blackmail game. Only Francis knew exactly what needed to be done: "In his windowless office in Phoenix, he began laying out his own long-range plans for getting ahead of the epidemic." (*ATBPO* p.232) He wanted an outside advisory group of immunologists and retrovirologists to guide the CDC. New-fangled retrovirologists — not old-fashioned virologists.

With his retroviral thinking cap on, Francis wanted to hone in on implacable retrovirus-spreading sexual behaviors of the gays: One of his almost salivating tough love memo's said, "I feel that to control AIDS we are obligated to try and do something to modify sexual activity. No doubt neither the fear of gonorrhea nor syphilis nor hepatitis B has decreased the number of sexual partners among homosexual men. *But fear of AIDS might.* [Emphasis mine] It seems mandatory for CDC to spread word of AIDS to all areas of the country. We have the network of VD clinics by which this word can be spread. Why not try?"(*ATBPO* p.233) Word certainly had no trouble spreading—and turning everything in its path into what I call Holocaust II. Thus, a biased, gay-obsessed presumption about the nature of AIDS was seamlessly stitched into the thinking and public health message right from the get-go. Every time the nature of the epidemic would be discussed, it would send a clear anti-gay message. Every time a public health warning about the epidemic would be given, it would repeat what I call the biased conventional "homodemiological" wisdom. If it was not consciously a big lie, it was a Big Mistake being promoted with the same effective propagandistic techniques. And over time the Big Mistake would evolve smoothly and inexorably into the Big Self-deception and the Big Lie.

Francis was so committed to his retroviral explanation of AIDS that he could not let any anomalous or contradictory data get in the way of his retroviral, venereal, and gay paradigm. He had created what Hannah Arendt might have called an "epidemiological image." He began to build an empire around his AIDS paradigm, firing off memos insisting that "as part of CDC's continuing pursuit of the cause of AIDS, a laboratory with retrovirus capabilities is necessary at CDC." (*ATBPO* p.266) He moved to Atlanta and assumed the title of "Lab Director for the AIDS Activities Office." A great time was about to be had by all.

The CDC bureaucracy that Francis had to deal with is portrayed in the Shilts book as unenlightened and slow to respond to the AIDS mensch. Historians will have to do some homework here and figure out if maybe there were some unsung heroes of insurgency at the CDC who actually took the correct measure of Francis and acted appropriately. Sabotage of the Francis agenda might in retrospect have been the work of unrecognized saints. Shilts portrays Francis as someone who was heroically willing to go outside legal channels to achieve his worthy (in his own visionary mind) goals. Francis was willing to spend money without congressional authorization. (Yes, AIDS now had its own Oliver North.) Francis was often so busy with his "AIDS activities" that he didn't have time to write up findings for publications. Why write up findings for publications when people were dying? This was an implacable gay behavior emergency. Not bothering to write things up is a chronically disturbing meme in the abnormal science of AIDS.

Francis is characterized as the voice of sanity compared to Shilts's portrayal of Robert Gallo, the scientist who will claim—with guns blazing—to have discovered the true AIDS retrovirus. There was a curious meeting in July, 1983 (two years after the first formal newspaper reporting of the sighting of the epidemic) at the CDC which "had been called to try to coordinate the search for the retrovirus responsible for Acquired Immune Deficiency Syndrome." (*ATBPO* p.349) Historians who like to know what people knew and when they knew it will chomp at the bit to figure out the prescience of *knowing* it was a retrovirus before they had found it. There will always be the whiff of phoniness about the search for a predetermined cause and that phoniness will certainly give birth to all kinds of conspiracy theories as historians excavate this somewhat hazy period at the CDC. God only knows what they will find.

Shilts's depiction of Gallo's vainglory and hair-trigger temper serve only to increase the number of halos floating above Don Francis's head. When Francis tries to recruit one of Gallo's assistants (also known as "flunkies"), Gallo goes ballistic, which is not surprising as the story about what really goes on in Gallo's lab will reveal later in the decade. The skeletons in *that* scientific closet are a Halloween unto themselves. The Gallo assistant who jumps ship receives the usual Gallo going-away gift for such an occasion: "I will destroy you," Gallo says to the man, according to Shilts. (*ATBPO* p.368)

Without understanding the disturbing implications, Shilts haplessly does a decent job of providing a snapshot of the political pressure that the CDC was under to name something (perhaps anything—and this retrovirus fit *that* bill) as the cause of AIDS: "James Mason, the CDC director, had a blunt directive for Don Francis on March 21 [1984] 'Get it done,' he instructed. In his scientific notebook, Don Francis wrote PRESSURE and underlined the word twice. The heat was on to resolve the 'AIDS' mystery, and Francis didn't have any doubts that the proximity of the presidential election motivated the unusual administrative concern." (*ATBPO* p.434)

Historians will have to ask themselves if the roots of the titanic mistake made on HIV, AIDS and HHV-6 was actually just driven by the politics of a presidential election year. Was it just that tragically simple? Did the dynamics of one presidential race give birth to the era of mistaken, sociopathic science that will refuse to correct itself for three decades? Did "Get it done!" lead, as night follows day, to Holocaust II?

Francis played pivotal role in the CDC's ultimately disastrous judgment that LAV, the retrovirus discovered by the French in AIDS patients, was the cause of AIDS. The bums-rush speed with which Francis moved from deciding it was the cause to creating inexorable public health policies based on his theory was stunning. Within a very short time frame there was an action agenda from Francis, and according to Shilts, "With the cause of AIDS found, scientists could now get on with the business of controlling the spread of the epidemic and finding a vaccine." (*ATBPO* p.409) Indeed. Given that the CDC could control *the information* about the spread of the epidemic (the manufactured Arendtian image, so to speak), they could certainly give the appearance of controlling the actual epidemic. That's how abnormal, totalitarian and ultimately sociopathic science, works.

Ironically, maybe one of the most important inadvertent contributions that Don Francis made to ultimately undermining the HIV/AIDS paradigm was his *inability* to create a model for "AIDS" by infecting monkeys with the retrovirus supposedly discovered by the French and Robert Gallo. This helped give birth to the first whistleblower of AIDS, retrovirologist Peter Duesberg, who used the failure to create an animal model as one of the arguments bolstering his growing doubts that the retrovirus was the real cause of AIDS. The health of those monkeys may have serendipitously saved all the people who heeded Duesberg's warnings about the questionable science of HIV.

Shilts portrays Francis as an earnest man committed only to furthering the interests of public health, the perfect foil to Robert Gallo. As Gallo appeared at a press conference with Secretary of Health and Human Services, Margaret Heckler, to claim that the cause of AIDS had been found, Saint Francis watched in horror: "After years of frustration, the announcement of the HTLV-III discovery deserved elation, Don Francis thought as he watched the live Cable News Network coverage of the Heckler press conference in the CDC's television studio with other members of the AIDS Activities Office. Instead, he felt burdened by the conflicts he saw ahead. The French were being cheated of their recognition and the U.S. government had taken a sleazy path, claiming credit for something that had been done by others a year before. Francis was embarrassed by a government more concerned with election-year politics than with honesty. Moreover, he could see that suspicion would play greater, not a lesser role in the coming 'AIDS' research. Competition often made for good science, Francis knew, lending an edge of excitement to research. Dishonesty, however, muddied the field, taking the fun out of science and retarding future cooperation." (*ATBPO* p.451) Sleazy paths? Dishonesty? Suspicion? The world hadn't seen anything yet.

Luckily for the health and civil liberties of the American people, Donald Francis, sooner rather than later "was beginning to feel beaten down." (*ATBPO* p.462) While others focused on a search for a treatment for "AIDS," Francis was itching to take it to the gay tribespeople and to "implement widespread voluntary testing for gay men."(*ATBPO* p.469) And gay men just couldn't wait until he got his hands on them. The "voluntary testing," of course, was based on his heterosexist notions of the epidemiology and virology of the disease. Francis penned a visionary nine-page program called "Operation AIDS Control" and his plan "employed the only two weapons with which health authorities could find the epidemic—blood testing and education." (*ATBPO* p.524) Luckily for the gay community, he never completely succeeded in getting the CDC into the full monty "control modality." But the early work of Francis succeeded in creating a paradigm that would help steer the AIDS agenda for three sociopathic decades, one that implied that the only way to control the epidemic was to find ways to intervene medically and social-engineeringly in the lives of gay people. If civil rights, demedicalization, and privacy had been spoils of gay liberation, they were now under direct threat from the public health vision presented by Francis and his colleagues. According to Shilts, "Francis drew his two circles. One circle represented men infected with the AIDS virus; the other men who weren't. The point of AIDS control efforts, he said should be to make sure that everybody knows into which circle they fit." (*ATBPO* p.549) Dante couldn't have drawn better circles for the gay community. You could also say it was the epidemiological equivalent of dividing and conquering.

To their credit, not all gay men were eager to split their community up into Don Francis's two vicious circles. For the majority of the gay community, who began to live their lives in the shadow of the two fraudulent circles, trusting in Francis's vision proved a huge mistake. By 2010, one study of gay men showed that the big circle had not been protected from the real epidemic by avoiding contact with the smaller circle. One study showed that 60% of all gay men were testing positive for HHV-8 the so-called Kaposi's sarcoma virus, originally a marker for AIDS. In terms of the AIDS-like illnesses not related to HIV, that would turn out to be the tip of the iceberg. Trusting white knights like Don Francis and believing in HIV did not save the gay community from the real epidemic. In fact, for many, that made it worse.

Even his boss, James Curran, was not quite willing to turn over the epidemic to the gung-ho Donald Francis. A disgruntled Francis eventually left the CDC to go work in the San Francisco Health Department. Shilts leaves us with the impression that the proactive Don Francis could have saved the world if only the system hadn't gotten in his way. Francis had warned the world but he "had only been beaten by the system, and because of that the disease had won." (*ATBPO* p.600)

A disease had definitely won, but not the one Francis thought he had been fighting while wearing his venereal and retroviral glasses—the ones with the heterosexist frames. That disease, of course was the HHV-6 pandemic which includes Chronic Fatigue Syndrome, autism, cancer, etc. The list goes on and on.

James Curran and the Really Identifiable Gays

"What a man sees depends on what he looks at and also upon what his previous visual-conceptual experience has taught him to see."

—Thomas Kuhn (*SSR* p.113)

The Centers for Disease Control's James Curran was one of the chief architects of the original AIDS paradigm. Curran had the perfect medical background for laying down the formative heterosexually-biased interpretations of the early data that epidemiologists gathered about the sick gay men who were thought to be the patients zero of a new supposedly gay epidemic. Jacob Levenson described Curran in *The Secret Epidemic: The Story of AIDS and Black America*: " . . . Jim Curran, the Chief of the CDC's Venereal Disease Control Division was tapped to head up a Kaposi's Sarcoma and Opportunistic Infection Task Force. Despite being short staffed and underfunded, the Task Force managed to bring together experts from diverse fields like virology, cancer, and parasitic diseases in addition to a small team of epidemiological intelligence officers, who were the agency's foot soldiers for disease prevention. . . . He had done quite a bit of work on hepatitis B with gay men in the 1970s, and he almost immediately suspected that he had a similar sexually transmitted and blood borne disease on their hands." (*The Secret Epidemic: The Story of AIDS and Black America*) And that suspicion paved the way for one of the biggest conceptual mistakes in the history of epidemiology.

According to Shilts's *Band*, when Curran saw the first reports on PCP in gay men, he wrote an odd note to one of his colleagues saying, "Hot stuff. Hot stuff." (*ATBPO* p.67) Shilts also described a rather revealing meeting at a subsequent CDC conference at which Curran was briefed on the sexual behavior of gay men by a chatty gay physician named David Ostrow. According to Shilts, "Ostrow mused on the years he had spent getting Curran and Dr. Jaffe [Curran's CDC colleague] acculturated to the gritty details of gay sexual habits. . . . Curran had seemed uptight at the start, Ostrow thought, but he buckled down to his work. Both Jaffe and

Curran were unusual in that federal officials rarely had any kind of contact with gays, and the few who did rarely wanted to hear detailed gymnastics of gay sex." (*ATBPO* p. 68) They clearly buckled down to their work a little *too* well. With their heterosexual sense of noblesse oblige (venereal division), these high-level clap doctors gone wild, set out to understand what the mysterious new gay epidemic was all about. Gay men would have run for the hills or hidden in basements if they had known what would result from the efforts of these two quick learners about "the gymnastics of gay sex" who were headed their way loaded for bear. The CDC's new experts in the joy of gay sex were now about to destroy the joy of gay sex.

Curran was married and the father of two children. Three days into what he thought was the sexually transmitted epidemic, he was examining gay patients and, already, according to Shilts, he "was struck by how identifiably gay all the patients seemed to be (*ATBPO* p.70) These gays were apparently *really gay*, not the plainclothes kind who could pass. According to Shilts, these gays "hadn't just peeked out of the closet yesterday." (*ATBPO* p.71) It may have been the perceived intense gayness of the first patients— the really gay ones—that resulted in Curran's huge, consequential mistake of erecting a mostly gay venereal epidemiological paradigm that would become the virtual thirty year hate crime against all gays, both the ones who could pass and the ones who were *really* gay. It wasn't just the patients who were strange. The strangeness of the people who had the disease would inspire a strange new kind of science, epidemiology and virology that was in essence "homodemiology." It was destined to make everything worse for gays and everyone else who had the bad luck of getting caught up in the CDC's paradigm. And that would ultimately even include members of the heterosexual general population. Otherwise known as epidemiological collateral damage.

Shilts tried to capture Curran's thought process when he wrote, "It was strange because diseases tended not to strike people on the basis of social group." (*ATBPO* p.71) He added, "To Curran's recollection . . . No epidemic had chosen victims on the basis of how they identified themselves in social terms, much less on the basis of sexual lifestyle. Yet, this identification and a propensity for venereal diseases were the only things the patients from three cities—New York, Los Angeles, and San Francisco—appeared to share. There had to be something within this milieu that was hazardous to these people's health. (*ATBPO* p. 71) Well, there certainly was something about to enter this "milieu" that would be extremely hazardous to these people's health, and that was Curran himself and his merry band of gay-sex-obsessed groupthinking epidemiologists who were about to hang the albatross of the venereal AIDS paradigm around the neck of the entire gay community.

When Shilts discussed Curran confronting "sociological issues" that were involved in the mysterious illness, it escaped Shilts that Curran and his associates *were themselves sociological (and political) issues* as they plopped themselves in the middle of the gay community (at a time when the community was most vulnerable and nearly hysterical) with all of their own peculiar heterosexual and heterosexist baggage. According to Shilts, "About a dozen staffers from all the disciplines potentially involved with the diseases volunteered for the working group. They included specialists in immunology, venereology, virology, cancer epidemiology, toxicology and sociology. Because the outbreak might be linked to the Gay Bowel Syndrome, parasitologists were called in. (*ATBPO* p. 71) The fact that any illness was labeled "Gay" should probably have been a red flag for the kind of heterosexist thinking that would soon be rolling across the gay community like a tsunami.

Once the guiding gay-obsessed premise was set, it was a matter of gay epidemiological garbage in and gay epidemiological garbage out. Questions with mistaken premises were about to lead the researchers and their medical victims down a deadly primrose path. Shilts summed up the basic direction of the inquiry: "Researchers also sought to determine whether the disease was indeed geographically isolated in the three gay urban centers. Did the detection of cases in the three centers make the patients appear to be only fast-lane gays because gay life tended toward the fast track in those cities? Was the disease all over gay America but in such low numbers that it had not been detected?" (*ATBPO* p. 81) Now we know, of course that there *was* indeed something else out there, but not just "all over gay America." Something wasn't playing by the rules of the CDC's gay-obsessed epidemiology. And that something was the very epidemiologically inconvenient Chronic Fatigue Syndrome epidemic

There is something almost laughable about the notion of Curran's CDC working group going out into the gay world and asking themselves what "new element might have sparked this catastrophe." (*ATBPO* p.82) One brand new element in the gay community that actually was the most significant spark for the coming catastrophe that was about to unfold was the CDC's own incompetence and heterosexist epidemiology.

Given the way AIDS would evolve into the kind of abnormal and sociopathic science that doesn't even require the usual rules of evidence, common sense, or logic, it is interesting that Curran *did* apply those old-fashioned rules early on when they were needed to build the venereal AIDS paradigm. Shilts wrote, "To prove an infectious disease, Curran knew, one had to establish Koch's postulate. According to this century-old paradigm, you must take an infectious agent from one animal, put it into another, who becomes ill, and then take the infectious agent from the second and inject it into still a third subject, who becomes ill with the same disease." (*ATBPO* p.105) Curran certainly tried to apply some semblance of the paradigm—or the logic of it anyway—when, by finding people who had AIDS often had slept with people who also had the disorder, he saw the links as a kind of epidemiological proof of transmission even though they weren't strictly speaking the fulfillment of the animal experimentation inherent in Koch's postulate. At least Curran knew the basic rules of science. Unfortunately, these very same rules would subsequently be thrown out the window to maintain the belief that the retrovirus eventually linked to AIDS was the one true cause of AIDS. Had those Koch's postulates been adhered to faithfully throughout the epidemic, we might be calling HHV-6 the virus of acquired immunodeficiency today and there might have been no Holocaust II or mysterious Chronic Fatigue Syndrome epidemic to write about.

The CDC, in an evolving and de facto manner, conducted something that could be called "the Atlanta AIDS/CFS public relations experiment" at the expense of everyone's health. What I mean by that coinage is a kind of postmodern public health political experiment in which rather than truly controlling an epidemic by being truthful and effective and scientific, the public health institutions of the CDC and the NIH tried to control and manipulate everything the public *knew* (and didn't know) about the epidemic of AIDS and CFS. It may have been quasi-innocent and simply the product of unrecognized sexual bias and old-fashioned self-deception when it started, but it evolved into something far more sinister and destructive. In the early days of AIDS, as described by Shilts, Curran was seemingly the embodiment of good-egg innocence when it came to the realization that it would be necessary for him to figure out some way to get the media's attention in order to increase public pressure for providing the funding the CDC needed for AIDS research. Unfortunately, the manipulation of the media by scientists or public health officials can—and did—have grave consequences for scientific, medical and epidemiological truth. In AIDS it became a kind of cancer that spread to the farthest reaches of public health.

In 1982 Curran appeared before a group of gay physicians in New York and told them "It's likely we'll be working on this most of our lives." (*ATBPO* p. 134) Historians one day will want to probe deeply into whether he knew anything that everyone else didn't know at that point. At the very least, it was as though he was an inadvertent prophet. He and his colleagues were indeed in the process of screwing things up for many generations to come. Curran's mistakes assured that his grandchildren's grandchildren will probably still be working on this problem. If they're not suffering from the myriad consequences of HHV-6 infections.

Shilts, in another moment of ironic journalistic naiveté, wrote this about Curran: "As a federal employee Curran had a thin line to walk between honesty and loyalty" (*ATBPO* p. 144) when he was describing the AIDS situation to Congress. Shilts notes that Curran could not ask Congress for money when he testified, "but he could nudge facts toward logical conclusions." (*ATBPO* p. 144) The nudging of facts would become an art form at the CDC over the next three decades and sometimes the facts that had to be nudged were so large they virtually had to be moved with bulldozers and the conclusions they were nudged towards were always more political than logical. One could almost faint from the irony of Curran telling Congress in 1982, "The epidemic may extend much further than currently described and may include other cancers as well as thousands of persons with immune defects." (*ATBPO* p. 144) Had he or his colleagues at the CDC recognized that cases of AIDS-like Chronic Fatigue Syndrome were simultaneously occurring all over the country, he would have been talking about millions (if not billions) of cases and he would not have had to play games with words to get Congress and the White House to do the right thing financially. One disturbing aspect of his manner of thinking was reflected in how Shilts summed up his testimony: "With death rates soaring to 75 percent among people diagnosed with GRID for two years, the specter of 100 percent fatality from the syndrome loomed ahead, he added." (*ATBPO* p.144) It would be nearly impossible to dial back on the distorted image of the epidemic he was presenting and frankly, dialing back on anything was something that the CDC (like the NIH) would turn out to be constitutionally unable to do. That, as we have said, is another sign that we are living in a period of totalitarian, abnormal, and sociopathic science.

Curran's peculiar attitude towards gays surfaced revealingly again when Shilts described his refusal to meet Gaetan Dugas, the unfortunate gay man who would be eternally scapegoated in the echo chambers of the media as the "Patient Zero" of the AIDS epidemic because he had supposedly slept with a number of the original AIDS cases: "Jim Curran passed up the opportunity to meet Gaetan, the Quebecois version of Typhoid Mary. Curran had heard about the flamboyant [flight] attendant and frankly found every story about his sexual braggadocio to be offensive. Stereotypical gays irritated Curran in much the same way that he was uncomfortable watching Amos n' Andy movies." (*ATBPO* p.158) One doesn't know quite where to begin on this one, except to note that Curran would be able to use his clap-doctor and gay-obsessed epidemiology to act on his feelings and beliefs about both stereotypical and non-stereotypical gays, and every other kind of gay in between. The way that Shilts described Gaetan Dugas should have been a warning to the whole gay community of what kind of medical and social treatment was in store for them: "Gaetan Dugas later complained to friends that the CDC had treated him like a laboratory rat during his stay in Atlanta, with little groups of doctors going in and out of his hospital room. He'd had his skin cancer for two years now, he said, and he was sick of being a guinea pig for doctors who didn't have the slightest idea what they were doing." (*ATBPO* p.158) Of course when those doctors eventually thought they *had* figured out what they were doing—that was precisely when they really didn't really have a clue about what they were doing. The Holocaust II era of the gay guinea pig had only just begun. The CDC's epidemiology would create a whole new gay stereotype. Curran's difficulty in getting researchers to come into the field was the fallout of the gay and sexual way the frightening disease had been framed for the public— something that might never have happened if the heterosexual Chronic Fatigue Syndrome cases had been included in the epidemiological and virological template for the epidemic.

It's amazing how many people seem to have been assigned credit (by different sources) for bringing (dragging?) Robert Gallo into AIDS research. Shilts has Curran on that Washington-slept-here list too, noting that he said to Gallo when he was receiving an award at a medical conference in 1982, "You've won one award. You should come back when you win another award for working on AIDS." (*ATBPO* p. 201) Bringing Gallo into the field was like putting a pair of retrovirus-obsessed eyeglasses over a pair of gay VD-obsessed eyeglasses and expecting to see the epidemic for what it was. Otherwise known as the blind recruiting the blind.

One of the more grimly amusing passages in Shilts's book concerns Curran's thought about the fears in the gay community that AIDS would result in gays being put into concentration camps: "Curran thought the train of thought was curious. After all, nobody had suggested or even hinted that gays should be in any way quarantined for AIDS. The right-wing loonies who might propose such a 'final solution' were not paying enough attention to the disease to construct the Dachau scenario. Still, it was virtually an article of faith among homosexuals that they should end up in concentration camps." (*ATBPO* p. 228) Silly gays. Frankly, who needed concentration camps or "the Dachau scenario" when you had CDC epidemiology. CDC epidemiology saved the country a load of money on barbed wire. And Holocaust I, where gays actually were made to wear pink triangles in real concentration camps—that was so 1940s.

One of the most unfortunate and tragically wrongheaded things about Curran is that, according to Shilts, he held his colleague Donald Francis "in awe, given Francis's international reputation for smallpox control." (*ATBPO* p.262) As one looks back at the circle jerk that also got Germany's Holocaust I going, one might hypothesize that all holocausts begin in passionate mutual admirations societies.

Something began to surface during James Curran's reign over AIDS at the CDC that bears close scrutiny by any enterprising historian interested in identifying the institutional roots of Holocaust II. In 1983, when Susan Steinmetz, an aide to Congressman Ted Weiss, visited the CDC in an oversight capacity, she was prevented from seeing files she automatically should have been able to audit as a representative of a Congressional Committee that had oversight responsibilities on health and the environment. According to Shilts, she was told by the then CDC Director William Foege, "she would not have access to any CDC files, and she could not talk to any CDC researchers without having management personnel in the room to monitor the conversations. The agency also needed a written, detailed list of specific documents and files Steinmetz wanted to see." (*ATBPO* p.292) Shilts reported that "Steinmetz was flabbergasted. What did they think oversight committees did? Their work routinely involved poring through government files to determine the truth of what the high-muck-a-mucks denied, and then privately talking to employees who, without the prying eyes of their bosses, could tell the truth. This was understood, she thought." (*ATBPO* p.292) What she didn't realize was that the CDC's de facto counterrevolution against science and the ideal of transparency in democratic processes had begun before her unassuming eyes and this would become business as usual at the clandestine CDC for the next three decades. The iron curtain of secrecy (de rigueur in all abnormal and sociopathic science) that would enable Holocaust II and the cover-up of the CFS and HHV-6 epidemic had descended.

While Steinmetz was just trying to find memos that would contradict the CDC's public posture that it had enough money to research the emerging epidemic of AIDS, without realizing it, she had stumbled onto the fact that the CDC had begun acting more like a government intelligence agency with vital national secrets—possibly even embarrassing ones—to keep, than a public health organization that was committed to truthful science and was accountable to the American people. In essence the CDC was showing that it wasn't above any of the legerdemain that any other part of the government was capable of. It was showing us that it was very much cut from the same cloth as the government gremlins that gave us Watergate and Vietnam. You could say that the CDC was perhaps the deepest part of the putative Deep State.

Steinmetz wanted to see files that pertained to budgets and planning, but she was bizarrely told that she couldn't see the files because they had patients' names in them and that violated patient confidentiality. It strained credulity to argue that patients' names were involved in organization budgets and planning. and in retrospect, it was a very lame excuse. This wouldn't be the first time in Holocaust II that a dishonest explanation with a fake concern and compassion for patients' welfare would be used by those in authority to stonewall the very people who were actually trying to *do* something about the welfare of patients. The CDC was already in a paranoid circle-the-wagons mode that characterizes abnormal and totalitarian science. According to Shilts, "The CDC personnel, who struck Steinmetz as peculiarly contentious, wanted to conduct their own review of the files before letting Steinmetz see them." (*ATBPO* p. 292) And "as another demand, the CDC insisted that before any interviews with CDC staff took place, the agency would screen questions that Susan Steinmetz put to scientists." (*ATBPO* p.292) On the eve of the HHV-6 catastrophe and Holocaust II, government science was going into the lockdown of abnormal, sociopathic science. Shilts wrote, "This is getting pretty strange, Steinmetz thought." (*ATBPO* p.292) Strangeness was but a puppy at that point.

This new emerging opposite world of public health and scientific duplicity and defensiveness didn't make sense to Steinmetz's colleagues back in D.C.: "On the phone, other oversight committee staffers in Washington confided that they had never heard of an agency so recalcitrant to Congress . . ." (*ATBPO* p.292) It got even worse for Steinmetz at the CDC in Atlanta when, on the second day of her oversight visit, she was told by the CDC manager who was handling her visit that her "presence would no longer be permitted in the CDC building and that no agency personnel would be allowed to speak to her." (*ATBPO* p. 293) The stonewalling and the lockdown were not confined to the CDC in Atlanta. Shilts reported that Steinmetz also faced new obstacles in her path when "The National Cancer Institute officials issued a memo demanding that all interviews with researchers be monitored by the agency's congressional liaison. At first the National Institutes for Allergy and Infectious Disease was cooperative, but then, in an apparent NIH-wide clampdown, information became difficult to excavate there as well." (*ATBPO* p.293) Science and public health in America were about to play the same kinds of political games that are played in totalitarian countries. Public health information was about to be totally controlled by the government.

Curran can himself take a great deal of personal credit for the HIV mistake. Shilts writes that "During the summer of 1983, Dr. James Curran had grown fond of citing the 'Willie Sutton Law' as evidence that AIDS was caused by a retrovirus. The notorious bank bandit Willie Sutton was asked once why he robbed banks, to which he replied, "Because that's where the money is." Curran, according to Shilts, would ask "'Where should we [at the CDC] put our money? . . . 'Where would Willie Sutton go? He would go with retroviruses, I think right now.'" (*ATBPO* p. 331) There is a revealing amount of cockiness and arrogance in Curran that remind one that pride goeth before a fall. But one Willie Suttonish thing was certainly true: retroviruses turned out to be exactly where the big money was for a number of dishonest and incompetent retrovirologists. And there would be serious consequences for anyone who noticed the AIDS had turned into an enormous confidence game.

It is fascinating to see Shilts catching Curran red-handed as he lies about the inadequate funding for AIDS. Publicly, Curran would say "we have everything we need," (*ARBPO* p.331) but Shilts was able to use the Freedom of Information Act to locate documents that "revealed that things were not so rosy at the CDC, and Curran knew it. Even while he reassured gay doctors in San Francisco, he was writing memos to his superiors begging for more money." (*ATBPO* p. 331) For anymore cognizant of the overwhelming mendacity that characterized just about everything concerning Holocaust II, it is especially disturbing to read Shilts's account of Curran's excuse: "'It's hard to explain to people outside the system,' he said. 'It's two different things to work within the system for a goal and talking to the people outside the system for that goal,' he said." (*ATBPO* p. 332) Curran was basically making the anti-transparency excuses people inside of the government always make for talking out of both sides of their mouths. It's too bad Shilts didn't consider the possibility *that this character trait was also reflected in the basic science and epidemiology of AIDS* that was being churned out by the CDC.

Curran got the venereal HIV/AIDS paradigm he and his colleagues wanted, the one that could be expected to materialize given his background. It wasn't surprising then, that he said in 1984, according to Shilts, "Gay men need to know that if they're going to have promiscuous sex, they'll have the life expectancies of people in the developing world." (*ATBPO* p.416) Actually, given the crazy toxic fraud-based treatments some gay men were going to be medically assaulted with, he was a true visionary.

As could be predicted, according to Shilts, "Jim Curran also viewed testing as essential to any long-term strategy in fighting AIDS." And so, the Pink Triangle medical apartheid agenda of testing and stigmatizing gays as HIV positive (or as an HIV risk group) began in earnest. And the gay community got specially tailored forms of communication from Curran. According to Shilts, "Curran was always cautious when he talked to newspaper reporters, fearful that his observations on the future of the AIDS epidemic might be fashioned into the stuff of sensational headlines, but he felt no inhibition with the gay community. Instead he felt his mission was to constantly stress the gravity of the unfolding epidemic." (*ATBPO* p.483) Of course, while he was giving the gay community the tough love, behind his epidemiological back was the looming HHV-6 spectrum and Chronic Fatigue Syndrome catastrophe, a biomedical event which was exponentially worse than anything his little team of jiggy clap doctors and pseudo-epidemiologists could possibly have imagined. Given that it was the CDC's AIDS paradigm that in essence scapegoated the gay community for what would turn out to be everyone's HHV-6 problem, it is the epitome of irony that according to Shilts, Curran thought that "the question was not if there would be a backlash against gays, but when. It might come soon. 'You should get ready for it,' he said." (*ATBPO* p.484) How does one prepare for a backlash against gays? Buy extra canned goods? Bake an extra quiche? It was certainly nice of him to give the gay community a heads up, but in truth, the pseudoscience, the incompetent fact-gathering implicit in ignoring the Chronic Fatigue syndrome cases that were occurring simultaneously, and the hard-wired homodemiology of the CDC, constituted a kind of epidemiological backlash *before* the backlash. Curran and his team needed only look in the mirror to see the kind of anti-gay values that could do far more mischief to the gay community than an army of right wing loons.

Journalist David Black caught some of the underlying psychological problems at the CDC in his book *The Plague Years*. He wrote, "In fact the CDC, like many physicians and scientists, seemed embarrassed by the gayness of the disease." (*TPY* p.57) We now know only too well in retrospect is that the best science and epidemiology cannot be conducted in an atmosphere of gay-sex-related embarrassment. Black quoted one CDC researcher as saying to a visiting gay activist, "This never would have happened if you guys had gotten married." (*TPY* p.57) When the activist asked if the researcher meant to each other, the researcher said, "To women." (*TPY* p.58) The CDC researchers conducted their epidemiology and science in an awkward atmosphere of antipathy to gays, surely not a fertile field for scientific objectivity. According to Black, when he asked Curran to explain exactly what he means by "'intimate contact' [between men] the phrase researchers kept using to describe the conditions under which the syndrome spread, he seemed uncomfortable, squeamish. He stammered and glanced anxiously around the room." (*TPY* p.58) If some of Jim Curran's best friends were gay, they had clearly done very little to make him comfortable with their sex lives. One suspects that most of Jim Curran's best friends were not gay.

One absolutely show-stopping moment in Black's rich little book is a criticism that was leveled at Curran: "He started making up these 'facts' from the data as he interpreted it,' said one unnamed gay critic of Curran." Who was that astute gay critic? Please stand up now, take your bow.

Mary Guinan's Missed Opportunity

Historians who want to trace the series of missteps that led to the HHV-6 pandemic and Holocaust II may benefit from taking a close look at a little known researcher at the CDC who played a curious role in both of the supposedly separate AIDS and Chronic Fatigue Syndrome epidemics. Her surprising inability to see an obvious link between the two syndromes may be one of the important seeds of the whole HHV-6 disaster. She is mentioned in both the Shilts history of the early AIDS epidemic and Hillary Johnson's *Osler's Web*, the definitive journalistic account of the CDC's bungling of the epidemic of facetiously-labeled Chronic Fatigue Syndrome.

According to Shilts, Mary Guinan worked for James Curran in the CDC's venereal disease division. She was the person who sent James Curran the first ill-fated report on the first cases of what would eventually be called "AIDS" in "homosexuals." With fellow VD chasers Harrold Jaffee and Curran, she shared the CDC AIDS Task Force's hoochie-coochie preoccupation with venereal diseases epidemiology. She helped impose the CDC heterosexist venereal groupthink on the emerging data of what would eventually be *gayified* epidemiologically into "Gay Related Immunodeficiency (GRID)."

Ironically, considering what turned out to be the role of HHV-6 in AIDS, Shilts reported that in 1981, "on a hunch, Guinan called a drug company that manufactured medicine for severe herpes infections. They told her about a New York City doctor who had been seeing . . . dreadful herpes infections in gay men." (*ATBPO* p.72) Shilts wrote that "Guinan was shaken by her investigation. She was accustomed to dealing with venereal diseases, ailments for which you receive an injection and are cured. This was different. She couldn't get the idea out of her head: There's something out there that's killing people. That was when Mary Guinan hoped against hope that they would find something environmental to link these cases together. God help us, she thought, if there's a new contagion spreading such death." (*ATBPO* p.72) One way that God certainly wasn't helping was by having a VD-obsessed doctor and her colleagues trying to comprehend a pandemic that wasn't, strictly speaking, venereal.

In Shilts's account of Guinan, seeing the epidemic through gay-obsessed lenses was a given. He wrote about one of her days in 1981: "It had been another typical day of gay cancer studies for Mary Guinan. She had wakened at 6 a.m to breakfast with gay doctors and community leaders and asked again and again, 'What's new in the community?' What new element might have sparked this catastrophe." (*ATBPO* p.82) It was just gay, gay, gay—24/7—for the AIDS Task Force. They simply couldn't wash the gay out of their hair. It was one of those times when every gay person should have checked to see whether they still had their wallets. Someone was about to sell them a gay epidemiological bridge.

As Shilts sympathetically presents Guinan, he inadvertently nails the whole CDC psychological and sociological bias problem: "Guinan felt helpless and frightened. This was the meanest disease she had ever encountered. She strained to consider every possible nuance of these peoples' lives." (*ATBPO* p.83) What she really meant was gay nuances of gay lives. It is supremely ironic that Shilts wrote, "The CDC, she knew, needed to work every hypothesis imaginable into the case-control study." (*ATBPO* p.83) *Every* hypothesis imaginable? Really? Not by a long shot. How about the hypothesis that these cases were just extreme versions of the Chronic Fatigue Syndrome cases that the CDC had been informed about? The un-gay cases.

The process of identifying the emergence of the epidemic in nongay drug users, as described in Shilts's book, makes it clear how gaycentric the thinking of the pioneers of the AIDS epidemiological paradigm was: "At the CDC there was a reluctance to believe that intravenous drug users might be wrapped into the epidemic, and the New York physicians also seemed obsessed with the gay angle, Guinan thought. 'He's said he's not homosexual but he must be,' doctors would confide in her." (*ATBPO* p.83) Everybody was becoming an expert on gayness in those days. Given the reluctance to even see connections in those cases of nongay drug-using outcasts, it should come as no surprise when years later anyone who saw the obvious connections between the epidemics of AIDS and Chronic Fatigue Syndrome was treated like they were strictly out to lunch. The AIDS paradigm was fatefully and messily intertwined with all the psychological baggage of sexual titillation and repulsion. (Hannah Arendt describes a similar phenomenon in the psychology of antisemitism.) If the CDC was unprepared psychologically to see drug users "wrapped into the epidemic," how about all the good clean living white heterosexuals with the AIDS-like permutations of the immune system that characterize Chronic Fatigue Syndrome? Can't go there.

Guinan's San Francisco trip with Harold Jaffe to interview AIDS patients and heterosexual controls also revealed the CDC mindset: "The CDC staffers could tell gay from straight controls by the way they reacted to the questions about every aspect of their intimate sexual lives. Heterosexuals seemed offended at queries about the preferred sexual techniques, while gay interviewees chatted endlessly about them." (*ATBPO* p.96) Oh those gays! A herd of chatty Cathies if ever there was one. Given the bias-laden epidemiology that this chattiness was about to imprison the gay community in, one is tempted to say that loose gay lips sank a proverbial legion of gay ships. If one were watching this on a screen in a movie theater, one would want to scream out to the clueless gay interviewees for their own sake, "For Heaven's sake, shut up!"

Guinan was one of the CDC researchers credited by Shilts with recognizing that hemophiliacs and blood transfusion recipients might ultimately also become victims of "gay pneumonia." She also was one of the first to worry about the AIDS infection possibilities of "semen depositors." (*ATBPO* p.132) Guinan cast a wide net: "No sooner had she convinced the CDC that intravenous drug users were indeed a category of GRID cases separate from gay men, then her field of investigations discovered the first reported GRID cases among prisoners and prostitutes." (*ATBPO* p.132) Unfortunately epidemiological net wasn't wide enough to catch the concurrent cases of AIDS-like Chronic Fatigue Syndrome. Also, unfortunately for her, she helped create the very consequential epidemiological urban myth of Patient Zero. She was the first person to come in contact with Gaetan Dugas the so-called gay Typhoid Mary who the CDC would turn into the "Patient Zero" or more appropriately, "Scapegoat Zero," of the epidemic depending on your point of view. He would become an icon for all the venereal *gaycentric* thinking down at the CDC.

In one of those amazing moments in Holocaust II in which a scientist comes so face-to-face with the truth but fails to see what is right before their eyes, Shilts reports that when Guinan was studying drug users, "blood sampling of the intravenous drug users also revealed that, although many were infected with cytomegalovirus, the viral strains were all different. This was strong evidence that the herpes virus had not developed some new virulent strain. No single strain emerged, lending further weight to Don Francis's hypothesis that a new virus, not CMV was at work." (*ATBPO* p.133) The CDC, in retrospect, was most likely eyeballing strains of an undiscovered virus that would be called HBLV when Gallo's scientists supposedly "discovered" it in 1986. It was subsequently named HHV-6. In retrospect it is pretty obvious that the CDC was looking at HHV-6 but thinking it was only CMV. (And those who *wanted to see a retrovirus* would have been especially predisposed *not* to see a new DNA virus like HBLV/HHV-6.)

It is interesting and perhaps revealing that Guinan and her colleagues could deal with the fact that the disease or syndrome *manifested itself differently* in gay men and drug users—presumably for reasons that would ultimately be figured out. But God forbid that anyone would subsequently suggest that even though there were differences in the manifestations of Chronic Fatigue Syndrome and AIDS that they were essentially manifestations of the same agent and the same pandemic. Distinctions were not turned into differences where drug users and gays were concerned, but where the gays with AIDS and the middle-class straights with Chronic Fatigue Syndrome were concerned, every distinction,—even the teeny-tiniest or most irrelevant kind—was immediately considered a dramatic how-dare-you-compare-these-apples-and-oranges difference. Such bogus thinking would be at the heart of the "Chronic Fatigue Syndrome is not AIDS" paradigm which would guide public health through the next three decades.

For all her good work Guinan was eventually rewarded with the position of assistant CDC director. Unfortunately for all the victims of HHV-6, what she did do at the CDC didn't have as much impact on the well being of the world as *what she did not do*. It was Guinan in 1985 who got a call from Dan Peterson, a former colleague and one of the two doctors who are credited with recognizing an outbreak of the absurdly named "chronic fatigue syndrome" in their Lake Tahoe practice. According to Hillary Johnson, "The two had become friends during a shared stint at the at the University of Utah hospital in Salt lake City in 1976." (*OW* p.31) Also, according to Johnson, "Peterson had frequently sought her counsel on different infectious disease cases; he had also struck her as a gifted diagnostician.' (*OW*. P.31)

Johnson reported that "Guinan listened as her former colleague described his Tahoe patients, her curiosity aroused by the possibility that this ailment, which three recent medical papers had described, was occurring in epidemic form. Previously, researchers had described it as a sporadic illness. She remembered too, that Atlanta clinician Richard DuBois [mentioned in my introduction] had made a presentation to agency staff on the malady early in 1983, even proposing that the new mono-like syndrome might be a second epidemic of immune dysfunction rising concurrently with AIDS." (*OW* p.31)

Did this lead Guinan serendipitously into a more complicated epidemiological vision of a variable epidemic that included both what was called "AIDS" and "Chronic Fatigue Syndrome"? Not on your life. These first CFS patients were not gay and not drug users. They were from medical practices that could be described as being devoted to folks who ride in the middle and front section of society's bus. Such stark social differences would make it of no consequence or interest that study after study would show one immunological and neurological similarity after another between AIDS and Chronic Fatigue Syndrome. Guinan had helped build a paradigm that was so gay, gay, gay and so socially radioactive that the links between AIDS and CFS would be willfully ignored, buried alive by denial, and through a kind of determined public health radio silence, for all intents and purposes, be covered-up big time.

Ignoring the obvious, Guinan sent the future "CFS" patients of America on one of the greatest medical wild goose chases in history. According to Johnson, she passed the Peterson cases on to Larry Schonberger, chief of the CDC's epidemiology within the Division of Viral and Ricketsial Diseases. Not surprisingly, Johnson reports that "Schonberger and his staff of epidemiologists had a mandate to monitor and occasionally investigate outbreaks of viral diseases, with the exception of AIDS, which by 1985 had been awarded a separate division and staff and more than half of the federal agency's entire annual research budget." (*OW* p.32) And so, because of Guinan's phone call and her very questionable judgment, CFS research headed down exactly the wrong road. Or, I should say, rabbit hole.

Had Guinan wisely directed the Lake Tahoe cases in the direction of the CDC's AIDS division back in 1985, there was still a chance that the political and medical apartheid of the "Chronic Fatigue Syndrome is not AIDS' paradigm and Holocaust II might not have been able to fully materialize. But AIDS had been so *gayified* and turned into such a sexual bogeyman and scarlet letter syndrome, that Guinan and everyone else at the CDC couldn't for the life of them admit that average (i.e. white heterosexual) Americans were coming down with any similar or related form of acquired immunodeficiency. Instead, those people were given the whitewash of a diagnosis of Chronic Fatigue Syndrome. Those good country people, to borrow a term from Flannery O'Connor, couldn't in a million years be suffering from something that had at one time or another been called Gay Cancer, Gay Plague, Gay Pneumonia, and Gay Related Immunodeficiency. After all, they weren't gay.

James Mason "Gets it Done"

"The sexual transmission of this illness, considered by most people as a calamity one brings on oneself, is judged more harshly than other means—especially since AIDS is understood as a disease not only of sexual excess but of perversity."
—Susan Sontag, *AIDS as Metaphor*

In its dark hours of 1983, the gay community needed nothing more than to have added to its tribulations the appointment of Dr. James Mason, a devout Mormon, to the office of Director of the Centers for Disease Control. They probably should have just counted their lucky stars that a member of the John Birch Society or Lyndon LaRouche himself wasn't appointed. According to Randy Shilts, "Until recently, he had served as state public health director for Utah. It was his friendship with conservative Utah Senator Orrin Hatch, the Chair of the Senate committee in charge of HHS, that had netted him the job as CDC director." (*ATBPO* p.399)

As we have already noted, James Mason uttered the fateful words ("Get it done!") that captured the whole pressure cooker environment that everyone working on AIDS operated in the first few years of the epidemic—both in and out of the government.

One useful thing that Mason *did do* was create an "AIDS Review Committee" to determine whether there were adequate resources for AIDS. According to Shilts, what the group discovered was that resources were being directed from other programs for AIDS: "Some 70 percent of the CDC's AIDS staffers were people diverted from other programs and not funded by federal AIDS appropriations." (*ATBPO* p.444) While the study ostensibly pointed to the need for more money for AIDS research, it also inadvertently showed *how easily the CDC could override the will of Congress* in terms of what actually got funded and therefore what actually got done. It was another disquieting bit of evidence that suggested something about the rogueish way the CDC did its own clandestine thing throughout the epidemic. What happened during Holocaust II shows that in some ways the CDC operates in some weird extralegal zone outside of the United States government and abides by its own rules. If nothing else, AIDS has taught us that public health can operate as a shadow government.

Mason seems to have been prone to the same kind of squeamishness toward all things gay as James Curran. Shilts reported that "Even Dr. James Mason was heard complaining that since he had become CDC director, he found himself talking to complete strangers about sexual acts he would not discuss with his wife even in the privacy of his own home." (*ATBPO* p.586) Time didn't seem to mellow or loosen up the good doctor because in 2009, according to a report by writer Jake Crosby on the Age of Autism website, James Mason was a member of the board of trustees for Evergreen International. According to Crosby, "Its mission is to help homosexuals 'diminish same-sex attractions and overcome homosexual behavior,' by the faith of Jesus." That a person with those kinds of beliefs played a key role in the development and implementation of the HIV/AIDS paradigm which launched and maintained Holocaust II should come as no surprise to anyone.

*

Everyone at the CDC must have been relieved and proud that sensational day in April of 1984 when Margaret Heckler took the stage wearing a very funky looking wig in Washington with Robert Gallo to announce that the virus that he basically had stolen from the French was the cause of AIDS and that treatments and vaccines would follow in short order. All the CDC's scapegoating and running around in obsessive gay circles for three years had paid off handsomely. It was one more successful chapter in the history of one of the greatest public health operations in the world. The problem, of course was, that their hard work and gay-obsessed heterosexist medical sleuthing had resulted in the biggest medical and scientific mistake in history. And there would be an inexorable price that we the people—gay and nongay—would all have to pay for that egregious error for many decades to come. I am, of course talking about the tragic multisystemic HHV-6 epidemic which I have continued to cover for more than a decade at HHV-6 University.

The Duesbergians

How a Brave and Brilliant Group of
Scientists Challenged the AIDS Establishment
and Why They Failed

Introduction

According to the *Holocaust Encyclopedia*, "The Nazis believed that male homosexuals were weak, effeminate men who could not fight for the German nation. They saw homosexuals as unlikely to produce children and increase the German birthrate. . . . Because some Nazis believed homosexuality was a sickness that could be cured, they designed policies to 'cure' homosexuals of their 'disease' through humiliation and hard work." The Nazis who were "interested in finding a 'cure' for homosexuality" developed a "program to include medical experimentation on homosexual inmates of concentration camps. These experiments caused illness, mutilation and yielded no scientific knowledge."

I refer to what happened to gays during this period as "Holocaust I." According to the United States Holocaust Memorial Museum website, "The severity of the persecution of homosexuals increased after the war's outbreak. In July 1940, Himmler directed that any convicted homosexual who 'seduced more than one partner' be sent to a concentration camp after completing his prison sentence to prevent the homosexual 'contagion' from spreading. After 1942, the SS embarked on an explicit program of 'extermination through work' to destroy Germany's 'habitual criminals.' Some 15,000 prisoners, including homosexuals, were sent from prisons to concentration camps, where nearly all perished within months."

It is also noted on the website that in the camps prisoners were forced to wear "marks of various colors and shapes which allowed guards and camp functionaries to identify them by category. The uniforms of those sentenced as homosexuals bore various identifying marks, including a large black dot" and later a "pink triangle."

The Holocaust Museum also notes, "After the war, homosexual concentration camp prisoners were not acknowledged as victims of Nazi persecutions and reparations were refused."

What I refer to as Holocaust I for gays was a part of what is traditionally referred to as "the Holocaust" or "the Shoah" which was a genocide in which six million Jews were killed. In the Holocaust the homosexuals were not the primary target. Their "crime" was not one of "racial inferiority" but rather for "behavioral inferiority." In Holocaust II they are the primary target.

In his book, *Life Unworthy of Life*, James M. Glass writes about the overlap of the medicalization of the Jews and the gays in Nazi Germany:

"It is critical not to underestimate the power of phobia in driving the perception of the Jew as bacillus translated into the public policy of sanitation and infection. Certain stories filtering back to Germany about the condition of the ghettos—the extent of disease, the deadly environment— added to the prevailing view of the Jew as bad blood. A similar attitude prevailed regarding homosexuality. In 1938, Reich Legal Director Hans Frank, who later became head of the General Government in occupied Poland, wrote that homosexuality 'is clearly expressive of a disposition opposed to the normal national community. Homosexual activity means the negation of the community as it must be constituted if the race is not to perish. That is why homosexual behavior in particular, merits no mercy.' In his diary Goebbels called homosexuality a 'cancerous disease.'"

What I call "Holocaust II" is the event that began in 1981, thirty-six years after the German forces surrendered to the Allies: the so-called "AIDS epidemic." As the publisher and editor-in-chief of a gay New York City newspaper called *New York Native*, I was destined to have a front row seat on the tragedy of Holocaust II as it unfolded. In the early years of the epidemic I focused my newspaper continuously on the epidemic and earned nearly universal praise for doing so when most of the media preferred to look the other way. In *Rolling Stone*, David Black said that we deserved a Pulitzer for our early coverage and Randy Shilts also gave it high marks in his bestseller, *And the Band Played On*. I have detailed that coverage and the entire history of my newspaper in my book, *The Chronic Fatigue Syndrome Epidemic Cover-up*.

While my newspaper's early coverage of the epidemic from 1981 to 1983 has been widely celebrated, our commitment to independent investigative and critical reporting about the epidemic eventually earned us the enmity of the government's medical and scientific establishment as well as the AIDS activist community. Things began to sour for us when we introduced our readers to the thinking of a molecular biologist named Peter Duesberg. Penned mostly by a writer named John Lauritsen, we gave extensive coverage to Duesberg's doubts about the HIV theory of AIDS. At first Duesberg was not sure what the cause of AIDS was, but he was certain it was not caused by a transmissible agent. As time went on, he began to promote a lifestyle theory of AIDS causation, pointing mainly to the use of recreational drugs.

Even though the scientific establishment did everything it could to debunk and silence Duesberg, he stood his ground and gained the support of a number of respected scientists and intellectuals who were also pilloried in one way or another for questioning the official AIDS dogma. I refer to his supporters and intellectuals who were inspired by him as "the Duesbergians." Even though there was a small army of Duesbergians, I have chosen to focus this book on four of the most prominent ones. Many of them had their own public and private theories about the causation of AIDS, but they generally had the same doubts about HIV as Duesberg. As the American government's official AIDS paradigm was increasingly carved into stone, Duesberg and the Duesbergians found themselves being called "AIDS denialists" who were a threat to public health. Some of the most powerful publications in the world mocked them, including *Science*, *Nature*, *The New York Times*, *The New York Review of Books*, and *The New Yorker*.

In addition to detailing Duesberg's critical thinking about the AIDS paradigm, John Lauritsen also reported on Duesberg's opposition to the use of some very toxic treatments for AIDS, most prominently, the drug called AZT which was being given to people who were diagnosed with AIDS or who had tested positive for HIV. Lauritsen's reporting on these matters are gathered in two important books, *The AIDS War*, and *Poison by Prescription*.

The *New York Native* became even more controversial in 1988 when I asked a writer, Neenyah Ostrom, to begin covering the relationship of AIDS to the mysterious emerging epidemic of what almost jokingly was called "chronic fatigue syndrome (CFS)." The obviously AIDS-like CFS epidemic had broken out concurrently with AIDS and seemed at first to mostly affect white heterosexual women. Ultimately, it was Ostrom's reporting in *New York Native* that was the biggest challenge to America's biomedical establishment, for it threatened to reveal that the entire AIDS paradigm was a house of cards and that the Centers for Disease Control was totally incompetent. Unfortunately for Duesberg and the Duesbegians, it also threatened to undermine the lifestyle paradigm of AIDS many of them were married to. Ostrom's reporting suggested that AIDS and chronic fatigue syndrome were actually two faces of a large pandemic caused not by the retrovirus HIV but by HHV-6, a DNA virus that was able to infect and harm many systems in the body and seemed to cause variable illnesses. Her reporting supported the notion that the Centers for Disease Control had defined the AIDS epidemic *too narrowly*, and as a result they had made one of the biggest errors in the history of science and medicine. The HHV-6 theory of AIDS challenged everything about the epidemic: the nosology, the virology, the mode of transmission, and the epidemiology. It meant that at best HIV was an exponentially stupid mistake or, at worst, a nefarious cover-up.

The picture of an HHV-6 epidemic that could endanger the health of the entire public in a variety of ways was terrifying. Given that it is no secret that public health officials seem to consider "panic control" part of their job description, it really is not shocking that the Centers for Disease Control has foolishly tried to keep a lid on information about the HHV-6 pandemic for more than three decades.

I have been studying this cockamamie political and medical event for more than half of my 67 years on this planet. It has been the center of my adult life. I sometimes think of it as an existential Rubik's Cube that I needed to be able to figure out as completely as possible. I think Hannah Arendt felt the same way about the Holocaust and Nazi Germany and it inspired her to write *The Origins of Totalitarianism*. You could say that much of what I have been writing about the AIDS epidemic constitutes my attempt to come to grips with the origins of what I call "totalitarian science," "sociopathic science," or "abnormal science." Thomas Kuhn's discussion of "normal science" in *The Structure of Scientific Revolutions* inspired my opposite-world label "abnormal science" for the pseudoscience of AIDS and its related biomedical issues. Both Kuhn and Arendt have been for me what Arendt refers to as "bannisters" in my attempt to think my way through the moral, political, and scientific disaster that is Holocaust II.

Much of my thinking about Holocaust II is contained in my book, *Iatrogenocide: Notes for a Political Philosophy of Epidemiology and Science*. In the introduction to that book I write, "I have concluded that what we think of as the epidemiology and science of AIDS are essentially a corrupted hard drive. Virtually all science and epidemiology conducted on that hard drive is false even though it has the appearance of being rational, progressive, and normal."

I have also come to the conclusion that science is inherently political and the politics of AIDS science are both antigay and racist. Antigayness and racism are hardwired into the epidemiology and pseudoscience of AIDS in the same way that antisemitism was hardwired into Nazi science. I came up with the term "homodemiology" to describe the kind of antigay epidemiology and science that blames diseases and epidemics on gays and cherry-picks or distorts data to support unwarranted and bigoted conclusions. ("Afrodemiology" is my word for the racist version of the same concept.) In the so-called AIDS epidemic, "public health" is the mask that homodemiology and Afrodemiology wear.

In many ways, my journey to these conclusions began with Peter Duesberg and the Duesbergians. Peter Duesberg and his courageous colleagues spoke out when the science of AIDS contained elements that just didn't make sense. They all took great risks in speaking out and they inspired people like me to think critically about every element of the AIDS epidemic. Ironically, the more critically I thought about the epidemic the more I saw that the members of the AIDS establishment were not the only ones who were getting the epidemic wrong. As right as they were about some things, I came to the conclusion that Duesberg and the Duesbergians did not fully grasp the mistaken nosology and epidemiology or antigay politics of the epidemic. Furthermore, they did not see the massive epidemic of HHV-6 that was driving an apocalyptic and variable epidemic in plain sight—one that included chronic fatigue syndrome, autism, multiple sclerosis, and many other "mysterious" illnesses.

For the last three decades, Duesberg and Duesbergians have been sucking up all the oxygen in the AIDS debate. Their arguments about HIV not being the cause of AIDS are cogent and it has been frustrating for them to watch the conventional wisdom triumph over truth. I think many of them are puzzled about their inability to wake up the intellectual community, the media, and the general public. I imagine many of them must lie in bed at night thinking "How can people be so stupid?"

I have written this book to celebrate their brilliance and bravery and to point out *what they got right*. I also discuss *what they got wrong* and explain why their mistakes prevented them from undermining a very corrupt AIDS establishment and thereby ending Holocaust II.

I hope they will accept my critique in the spirit of friendship and believe me when I say that, no matter what, I can never thank them enough for what they did.

Peter Duesberg

Half a Hero is Better than None

"As Max Weber put it, 'An exhaustive causal investigation of any concrete phenomenon in its full reality is not only impossible, it is simply nonsense.' Epidemiologists know this and do not attempt to include all causal factors in their analyses. They select some causes and omit others. Since the epidemiologist must, however, employ some criteria in the selection process, whether consciously or not, the final roundup of causes is never neutral. It necessarily reflects both the (human-made) rules of epidemiology and the values and assumptions of the person selecting the cause. The list probably reproduces many elements of the dominant political ideology as well, if only because the language we use to describe reality is so heavily influenced by the interests of powerful groups."

—Sylvia Noble Tesh,
Hidden Arguments: Political Ideology and Disease Prevention Policy (Page 68)

To say that the achievement of Peter Duesberg is a glass half-full should never be seen as damning with faint praise. Unflappable, imperfect Peter Duesberg heroically changed the course of the AIDS epidemic and history itself by his actions and part of his personal tragedy is that he could have changed it even more if he had looked deeper and been more critically attentive to the politics of the Centers for Disease Control's heterosexist epidemiology.

In the introduction to his 1987 interview with Duesberg, John Lauritsen wrote, "Peter Duesberg came to the United States about 20 years ago from Germany. He is professor of Molecular Biology at the University of California in Berkeley. It is because of his interest in retroviruses, on which he is an authority, that he became involved in questioning the 'AIDS virus etiology.'" (*The Aids War* p.47)

In that interview Duesberg argued that HIV could not be the cause of AIDS because of "the consistent biochemical inactivity of the virus." (*AW* p.47) He told Lauritsen that "Even in patients who were dying from disease, the virus is almost undetectable, while RNA synthesis is essentially not detectable, (*AW* p.47) Duesberg also said, "So that is one of the key arguments, and there is no exception to the rule that pathogens in order to be pathogenic have to be active." (*AW* p.48) He insisted, "very few potentially susceptible cells are ever infected, and those that are infected don't do anything. The virus just sits here." (*AW* p.48)

Duesberg also argued that the long latency period of the disease was "a very suspicious signal that the virus is unlikely to be solely the direct cause as they claim." (*AW* p.48) He pointed out that retroviruses "are the most benign viruses that we know" and "they can remain in the cell in latent form." (*AW* p.49) And most damning of all to the HIV hypothesis, according to Duesberg, was the fact that "When AIDS is diagnosed, they say that now it's possible for the disease—but the virus is not doing any more than it had done before when there were no symptoms of the disease." (*AW* p.49) Duesberg concluded that the presence of antibodies to HIV was proof that the virus had been neutralized and asserted that it was "a gross injustice to discriminate against anyone on the basis of having antibodies." (*AW* p.50)

One of the most noble aspects of Duesberg's AIDS criticism and whistleblowing on the HIV mistake (or fraud) issue was his extraordinary—almost visionary—sensitivity to the damage it was going to do to the health and liberties of those who were victimized by it. In general, the people he argued with, those who benefited financially and professionally from the HIV hypothesis, had a rather cold and cavalier attitude toward the effect their brilliant ideas often had on the minorities who were affected. (They certainly never seemed to ask themselves what the consequences would be if *they* were wrong.)

Duesberg deserves credit for being one of the first people to realize (without saying as much) that the HIV/AIDS theory was an instance of what I've called "abnormal science." One of the wittiest men engaged in the AIDS issue, he could often find the humorous absurdities implicit in the HIV theory. When HIV was called a "slow virus," he said, "There are no slow viruses, only slow scientists." In public forums, he always presented his opinions in a collegial manner, but he was also always capable of leaving his opponents hemorrhaging from a cutting sarcasm presented with deadly charm. It may have been the fact that he verbally earned the role of the alpha intellect in any professional gathering that inspired both envy and vengeance from his powerful HIV establishment opponents. They were often simply intellectually outclassed, even if they held all the money and the political cards. Nothing rattles totalitarian science more than a clever and steadfast nontotalitarian scientist.

If Duesberg suffered from any deficits in the area of judgment, it may have been an inability to imagine a different AIDS epidemic caused by a dynamic, multisystemic virus like HHV-6 (and its family) which could manifest itself in a variety of surprising ways (like AIDS, chronic fatigue syndrome and autism) depending on other factors. Duesberg told Lauritsen, "AIDS is a condition which includes so many parameters that it's almost inconceivable to define a simple pathogen as the cause, considering the diverse patterns of the disease." (*AW* p.52) Duesberg didn't think outside the box of the CDC's nosology or epidemiology. He never considered the possibility that the CDC had missed a whole world of undetected nosological and epidemiological data (like the data from the chronic fatigue syndrome epidemic) that would have completely changed the picture of the disease's patterns. And the idea that there might be something in the world that could be called a multisystemic virus like HHV-6 which *could* cause many different patterns of disease, was simply not on his radar.

At the time that Lauritsen first interviewed Duesberg—in 1987—Duesberg remained a bit of an agnostic on what was actually causing AIDS, saying, "We haven't excluded anything" and "I really wonder what it could be." (*AW* p.53) Compared to where he would end up, he was a demure etiological virgin at that point. He was only beginning to consider the role of recreational drugs as a possible cause saying, "I'm really just guessing here, but I think this is where more research should be done." (*AW* p.53)

Unfortunately, as time went on Duesberg seems to have been encouraged or even pressured by some of his colleagues to take a stronger public stand on what he thought actually *was* the cause of AIDS and he became far less tentative and open-minded, passionately adding to his anti-HIV gospel a seemingly unshakable conviction that recreational drugs explained AIDS in gay men. Regardless of its merits, such a position immediately lost him the readymade constituency of the gay community who seemed to have been invited by Duesberg and his followers to be exonerated for a transmissible infection only to be convicted as a group in an alternative fashion for having a unique gay (and—let's not forget—criminal) drug-taking lifestyle. With some notable exceptions, Duesberg walked into a big gay "thanks but no thanks." He had jumped the gay shark. It was a tragic development for both parties, because politically, Duesberg really needed gay supporters to help him challenge the mistaken HIV hypothesis, which he felt was unfairly threatening their liberties and health of the gay community. He was the enemy of the gay community's determined CDC/NIH enemy, but he wasn't perceived as its friend. By rejecting Duesberg's half-a-glass of truth about the virus, the gay community ended up in the open arms of the AIDS establishment and crusading public health authorities complete with all the goodies they had in store for their willing, eager and all too compliant patient population.

Peter Duesberg detailed his argument about the nature of the AIDS epidemic and his struggle with the AIDS establishment in his book, *Inventing the AIDS Virus*, which was published by Regnery Publishing in 1998. In the publisher's preface, Alfred Regnery notes, "AIDS is the first political disease." In his acknowledgments, Duesberg wrote, "I extend my gratitude to my most critical opponents in the AIDS debate, who have unwittingly provided me the great volume of evidence by which I have disproved the virus-AIDS hypothesis and exposed the political maneuverings behind the war on AIDS." (*IAV* p.x)

Duesberg's book could be used as a primary text if college courses are ever given on the politics, sociology, and psychology of what I call "abnormal science." He fleshes out many parts of his argument against the HIV theory of AIDS causation already mentioned in his 1987 interview with Lauritsen. While Duesberg is often thought to be someone who encouraged the rethinking of the AIDS issue, the book supports the notion already mentioned that, in reality, he actually *never went far enough*, never really did a true radical rethinking of AIDS because he works with a tacit acceptance of the basic epidemiological premises and "facts" provided by the CDC and the HIV/AIDS establishment. By leaving their paradigm's "factual" assumptions standing, he ultimately jeopardized his own analysis. Duesberg's critical tact was to take the "facts" as they were provided by the CDC and to try and poke holes in their etiological logic by showing how they failed to successfully make predictions about the course of the epidemic or by arguing that the facts as given by the CDC contradicted other formally known (hence, published) facts. The problem was that AIDS involved ground zero nosological and epidemiological definitions of what an AIDS case actually was, and *if* that definition had, at the very beginning of the epidemic, been distorted by evidence that had been cherry-picked, or had been ignored because of political blinders, then there was a good chance that Duesberg—even with his superb skills of logic and reason— was trapped in an pseudoscientific funhouse of "garbage in garbage out." Saying the CDC mistakenly linked the wrong virus to cases of AIDS begs a question: And what if the CDC completely got the definition of AIDS cases wrong to begin with? Or, more troubling, that what the CDC thought were epidemiological apples and oranges were really all apples or all oranges.

Duesberg never illuminated *all* of the fundamental possibilities of what could have gone wrong nosologically and epidemiologically. Duesberg was in a Donald Rumsfeld situation where he didn't know what he didn't know.

Duesberg worked with the epidemiological predictions the AIDS authorities were giving him and tried to show that when the predictions based on them did not work out, they reflected poorly on the credibility of the HIV theory. He argued, "Officials have continually predicted the explosion of AIDS into the general population through sexual transmission of HIV, striking males and females equally, as well as homosexuals and heterosexuals, to be followed by a corresponding increase in the rate of death. . . . In short, the alleged viral disease does not seem to be spreading from the 1 million HIV-positive Americans to the remaining 250 million." (*LAV* p.5)

Duesberg's logic brilliantly skewered the CDC's notion that AIDS was an equal opportunity disease. But again, one has to note that the one caveat he didn't acknowledge was that if the CDC's definition of what an AIDS case was *turned out to be dead wrong*, then all bets were off about correlated and potentially causative factors. Just debunking the logic behind the weak correlation of putative AIDS cases with HIV was not the same as debunking the notion of *some fundamentally different kind of AIDS epidemic* still occurring, not only in the gay community, but also in some form in the general population. If, at the very basic level of defining what a case is and what a case isn't, profound mistakes had been made, then one couldn't really know where the disease was and where it wasn't. And then the issue of HIV not being the cause of what was being called AIDS would, in that case, be *totally beside the point*. If anything, the HIV mistake should have made people wonder if those in charge at the CDC had gotten something even more profoundly wrong in the initial working definition of AIDS which subsequently was carved in stone thanks to the totalitarian scientific culture that protected it.

Insofar as Duesberg recognized that it all just didn't add up, he graciously performed a great humanitarian service over and over again by telling the world that as long as the HIV establishment was in charge of AIDS we were essentially trapped in a realm of unreliable and untrustworthy pseudoscience where people were going to get hurt. And luckily, for three decades, at great personal expense, Duesberg valiantly refused to shut up. Perplexed, Duesberg wrote, "Something is wrong with this picture. How could the largest and most sophisticated scientific establishment in history have failed so miserably in saving lives and even in forecasting the epidemic's toll?" (*IAV* p.5) Ironically, given that Duesberg himself was blind to what turned out to be the CFS epidemic and HHV-6 spectrum catastrophe, the premise of his rhetorical question turned out to be a tragic understatement.

Duesberg's suggestion about what should be done reinforces the notion that his call to a reassessment of AIDS and HIV just wasn't intellectually radical or fundamental enough. Duesberg's prescription for the problem was that "Faced with this medical debacle, scientists should re-open a simple but most essential question: What causes AIDS?" (*IAV* p.6) Again, it was not really a radical return to epidemiological ground zero. A return to ground zero would have involved asking if the epidemiological common immunological denominator that determined what a case actually was itself needed to be audited by looking closely—and in an immunologically sophisticated manner—*at the entire population*. Duesberg was like an accountant who looks at the books for discrepancies, but never goes into the warehouse to see if what's there matches the inventory numbers. His due diligence only went so far. The definition of AIDS was on the books and unfortunately, taken at face value by Duesberg. It didn't necessarily match what was actually going on in doctor's offices all over America and it didn't necessarily reflect the actual disaster that was occurring in the immune systems of the entire American population. There was a whole immunologically-challenged world beyond the CDC's published data and the peer-reviewed papers Duesberg used to play "gotcha" with the CDC's facts, logic, and conclusions.

There was an interesting groupthink bias in Duesberg and many of his followers, most of whom were heterosexual—some emphatically so. Not surprisingly, their notion about what was wrong with AIDS etiology *was always biased in the direction of heterosexuals being less (or not at all) at risk for AIDS* as a result of the CDC's scientific errors. Sometimes one got the uncanny notion that Duesberg and his followers were whistling heterosexually in the dark, engaged in trying to convince themselves that *they as a group* were safe from the "gay lifestyle" epidemic. Ironically, considering their apparent need for personal immunological safety, though, is the fact that *if* the CDC was wrong then all bets about their safety could have been off and the actual level of risk could have gone the other way. *They could have been in more, not less danger.* But that possibility never seemed to consciously dawn on them, and their AIDS dissident movement, in all its forms, seemed bent on making sure that it never did. They created a kind of dissident groupthink that made them odd bedfellows with the mostly white male heterosexual

HIV establishment who also could absolutely not let themselves see the connection between AIDS, chronic fatigue syndrome, HHV-6, and ultimately the simmering HHV-6-related autism disaster.

Duesberg got a lot of things right and a lot of things sort of right. He was right when he wrote, "Without going back to check its underlying assumptions, the AIDS establishment will never make sense of its mountain of data." (*LAV* p.6) He didn't quite get it right when he concluded, "The single flaw that determined the destiny of AIDS research since 1984 was the assumption that AIDS is infectious. After taking this wrong turn scientists had to make bad assumptions upon which they have built a huge artifice of mistaken ideas." (*LAV* p.6) Duesberg very simply failed to notice the fundamental wrong turn that was made before *that* wrong turn. He never considered the possibility that if the definition of AIDS itself was wrong, the corrected definition just might support the notion of an infectious epidemic and a virus-AIDS hypothesis, *just not the mistaken HIV one.*

The great thing about Duesberg—for students of what I've called homodemiology or heterosexist epidemiology—is that he criticized the logical absurdity of what I call GRID-think, (Gay-related immune deficiency) which is in part the rather superstitious and bigoted notion implicit in HIV epidemiology that *viruses know intuitively who gays are* so they can choose to infect them and only them. Unfortunately, Duesberg built his own quasi-GRID-think drug-and-lifestyle-paradigm on a similar reality-challenged premise by saying that something non-infectious must explain an epidemic confining itself mainly to a risk group. By pointing out the logical absurdity of a virus limiting itself to one group of people, he opened the way for a more radical critical political rethinking about what was going on in the CDC's epidemiology that he seemed unprepared to do himself. He started the job, but homodemiological and sociological analysis had to finish it. Blaming lifestyle factors of gays was just another not-very-great correlation fingered as causation, generating an alternative scapegoating epidemiology of blaming the victims for what turned out to be the HHV-6 spectrum catastrophe. Unfortunately, Duesberg exposed one wild goose chase and started another one when he wrote, "The only solution is to rethink the basic assumption that AIDS is infectious and is caused by HIV." (*LAV* p.7) The only solution? Well, not exactly.

Duesberg's book will always be an important source for anyone who wants to understand the evolution of the AIDS mistake, even if Duesberg's own theory turned out to be wrong. Most importantly, Duesberg details just how abnormal and nearly psychotic the whole scientific process of AIDS was and his work supports the argument that something with a totalitarian *je ne sais quoi* was unfolding in the name of AIDS science.

The very manner in which HIV was announced in 1984 as the probable cause of AIDS, according to Duesberg's account, was scientifically deviant: "This announcement was made prior to the publication of any scientific evidence confirming the virus theory. With this unprecedented maneuver, Gallo's discovery bypassed review by the scientific community. Science by press conference was substituted for the unconventional process of scientific validation, which is based on publications in the professional literature. The 'AIDS virus' became instant national dogma, and the tremendous weight of federal resources were diverted into just one race— the race to study the AIDS virus . . . . The only questions to be studied from 1984 on were how HIV causes AIDS and what could be done about it." (*IAV* p.8)

At that point in time, Duesberg noted that "serious doubts are now surfacing about HIV, the so-called AIDS virus . . . . The consensus on the virus hypothesis of AIDS is falling apart, as its opponents grow in number." (*IAV* p.8) At that moment Duesberg still seemed optimistic, as AIDS seemed to be taking place in the good faith universe of normal science which was open to change and paradigm shift. Unfortunately, because he was blind to the heterosexist sociological issues underpinning AIDS, he was incapable of perceiving the unmovable backstage anti-gay epidemiological values that were controlling the public health agenda and polluting the science. He couldn't see that it wasn't just a matter of the practitioners of this deviant science were digging in professionally; the whole homodemiological culture was dug in, which was far more formidable than anything Duesberg could have imagined. The political consensus about the etiological nature of "AIDS" was not a just stone in the road of scientific process. Peter Duesberg had found his way into abnormal science's opposite world.

As a paradigm that was supposed to capture people's imagination and cause a major shift or Kuhnian conversion—or visual gestalt-shift—from one consensus to another, Duesberg's paradigm was nearly dead on arrival. If he had simply taken his stand as a dean of retrovirology and just left the cause of AIDS up in the air and concentrated on demolishing the HIV theory once and for all, the HHV-6 catastrophe and what I call "Holocaust II" might have been stopped in their tracks.

Duesberg charged that the CDC's paradigm was "ineffective" and that "public fear was being exploited." (*IAV* p. 9) From his perspective, the public was being told the problem was bigger than it actually was. True, public fear was being shamelessly exploited, but *not in the way Duesberg thought*. By framing the epidemic in an anti-gay manner, public fear of gays, society's sexual outsiders, *was* being manipulated to hide the painful truth about the public's risk of developing a complex form of immunodeficiency or dysfunction. The public was being provided with what Daniel Goleman called "a vital lie." A terrified public, to the great detriment of its future health was getting the reassuring heterosexist pseudo-facts about "AIDS" it wanted to hear with the gay community losing what I call its *epidemiological human rights* in the process. And again, ironically, Duesberg and the Duesbergians had their own set of heterosexist concoctions that were *even more reassuring* to the heterosexual general population. And wrong. Both the CDC paradigm and the Duesberg paradigm misled a clueless and anxious public.

Duesberg's shock at the nature of what was going on is exactly why a formal theory of abnormal or totalitarian science is required to comprehend and illuminate the AIDS era, just as the concept of totalitarianism was required to understand the Hitler and Stalin eras. Duesberg asks a big, ugly, rhetorical question: "How could a whole new generation of more than a hundred thousand AIDS experts, including medical doctors, virologists, immunologists, cancer researchers, pharmacologists, and epidemiologists— including more than half a dozen Nobel Laureates—be wrong? How could a scientific world that so freely exchanged all information from every corner of this planet have missed an alternative explanation for AIDS?" (*IAV* p.9) Too bad he didn't ask how the exact same crowd could not see the chronic fatigue syndrome epidemic for what it was. Ditto for HHV-6 and its insidious spectrum.

Again, Duesberg's answer to his own question was that AIDS had been misclassified as an infectious illness and his theory rested on the notion that "the premature assumption of contagiousness has many times in the past obstructed free investigation for the treatment and prevention of a non-infectious disease—sometimes for years, at the cost of many thousands of lives." (*IAV* p.10) Duesberg was setting the terms of the twenty-five-year debate between the mainstream AIDS establishment and what became popularly known as the AIDS dissidents, or the Duesbergians. This unfortunate dichotomy set the course for the wrong kind of debate, a contest between HIV and Duesberg's non-infectious drug lifestyle hypothesis, leaving out the possibility that there might be a dynamic infectious agent *other than HIV* that did indeed fit the causation criteria of a redefined AIDS epidemic. No space was left in the debate for something like a new multisystemic virus such as HHV-6, which was capable of causing an epidemic of a more broadly defined variable illness. Duesberg asserted HIV "could be the most harmful of . . . fatal errors in the history of medicine if AIDS proves to be not infectious." (*IAV* p.10) Of course, if AIDS was incorrectly defined and a dynamic viral agent other than HIV was spreading *silently and exponentially* while the false Duesbergian debate sucked up all of intellectual and scientific oxygen in the debate on AIDS, the harm could have been exponentially worse. And it was.

In order for abnormal or totalitarian science to hold sway over a society for a long period of time, it must have ample cooperation from both the scientific and media communities and the Duesberg story provides evidence that such was the case in AIDS. To explain how the media was continuously kept in its subservient place during the AIDS debacle, he quotes reporter Elinor Burkett of *The Miami Herald*: "If you have an AIDS beat, you're a beat reporter, your job is every day to go out there, fill your newspaper with what's new about AIDS. You write a story that questions the truth of the central AIDS hypothesis and what happened to me will happen to you. Nobody's going to talk to you. Now if nobody will talk to you, if nobody at the CDC will ever return your phone call, you lose your competitive edge as an AIDS reporter. So it always keeps you in the mainstream, because you need those guys to be your buddies . . . ." (*IAV* p.388)

Duesberg insists that the very defensive and insular AIDS scientific establishment was determined to "confine the debate to scientific circles." (*IAV* p.389) He quotes a rather shocking threat from the de facto AIDS Czar, Anthony Fauci, who said, "Journalists who make too many mistakes, or who are sloppy are going to find that their access to scientists may diminish."(*IAV* p.384) In a totalitarian world of homodemiology and abnormal science the definition of "sloppy" will be that which contradicts the powers that be. Question AIDS and you will need to look for a new career. (Given the degree to which AIDS science often looks like a big unmade bed, it's amusing to hear Fauci say the word "sloppy" with a straight face.)

Duesberg also quotes two of the powerful, public-relations-savvy virologists who suggested another tactic for dealing with Duesberg and the critics of the HIV establishment: "One approach would be to refuse television confrontations with Duesberg, as Tony Fauci and one of us managed to do at the opening of the VIIth International Conference on

AIDS in Florence. One can't spread misinformation without an audience."
(*IAV* p.39) There's nothing in Thomas Kuhn's theories about the process
of normal science about deliberately denying one's critics an audience, or
denying the public exposure to scientific second and third opinions.

One of the more outrageous moments in his book occurs when
Duesberg writes, "Based on an anonymous source, key officials of the
United States government specifically engineered a strategy for suppressing
the HIV debate in 1987 while Duesberg was still on leave at the N.I.H. The
operation began on April 28, less than a month after Duesberg's first paper
on the HIV question appeared in *Cancer Research*, apparently because several
journalists and homosexual activists began raising questions." (*IAV* p.32) A
memo about Duesberg's critique of the HIV theory was sent out from a
staffer in the Office of the Secretary of Health and Human Services: "This
obviously has the potential to raise a lot of controversy (If this isn't the
virus, how do we know the blood supply is safe? How do we know
anything about transmission? How could you all be so stupid, and why
should we ever believe you again?) And we need to be prepared to respond.
I have already asked N.I.H. public affairs to start digging into this." (*IAV*
p.390) This is an extremely important memo from the point of view of
future what-did-they-know-and-when-did-they-know-it histories that try to
fathom all the government's motivations throughout this scientific and
political disaster. It shows how clearly at least one person in the
government could see the potential dire consequences for the government
of being wrong about HIV. Somebody knew *exactly* what was at stake.

In his book, Duesberg gives a number of examples of the media
seeming to have been pressured by the HIV establishment *not to cover the
story of the controversy*. According to Duesberg, "The MacNeil Lehrer News
hour sent camera crews to do a major segment on the controversy. But
when the . . . broadcast date arrived, the feature had been pulled.
Apparently AIDS officials had heard of its imminent airing and had
intercepted it." (*IAV* p.392) Television shows on Duesberg involving Good
Morning America on ABC, CNN, Italian television, and Larry King Live
met with a similar fate.

According to Duesberg's book, he "appeared on major national
television only twice. The first time was on March 28, 1993 on the ABC
magazine program *Day One*. Even in this case, according to the producer,
Fauci tried to get the show canceled days before broadcast.' (*IAV* p.393)
When Duesberg was interviewed for *Nightline*, he ended up only being given
a small amount of air time and Fauci showed up and was given the lion's

share of the show to make the HIV establishment's case. And Duesberg fared no better overseas. The British medical and public health establishment greeted a pro-Duesberg program with "stern condemnations" and subsequently the British press "turned around and began criticizing the program." (*IAV* p.323)

One of the most interesting moments of censorship occurred at the highest level of government when "Jim Warner, a Reagan White House advisor critical of AIDS alarmism, heard about Duesberg and arranged a White House debate in January 1988." (*IAV* p.394) Duesberg writes, "This would have forced the HIV issue into the public spotlight, but it was abruptly canceled days ahead of time, on orders from above." (*IAV* p.394)

Duesberg didn't fare much better with the print media. He notes that *The New York Times* had written about him only three times in the first seven years of the controversy and all of it was negative. The same kind of treatment was doled out by *The Washington Post* and "the *San Francisco Chronicle* intended to cover the story, until it encountered opposition from scientists in the local AIDS establishment." (*IAV* p.394) Even the countercultural or alternative press could not be counted on to give the controversy balanced or independent-minded coverage. Duesberg reports, "In 1989 *Rolling Stone* had commissioned a freelance writer from New York to write a Duesberg article, but then canceled it during the interview with Duesberg in his lab." (*IAV* p.395) Both *Harper's* and *Esquire* killed articles that had been commissioned on Duesberg during the same period. The media was essentially acting as an enabler of the culture of abnormal or totalitarian science.

Even more evidence that AIDS was a manifestation of abnormal science can be found in the way that Duesberg experienced censorship from formerly adoring scientific circles and experienced roadblocks to having his ideas and criticisms presented in the professional scientific literature. Duesberg writes, "Robert Gallo and some other scientists began refusing . . . to attend scientific conferences if Duesberg would be allowed to make a presentation." (*IAV* p.396) During the same period Duesberg rarely was "invited to retrovirus meetings and virtually never to AIDS conferences, despite seminal contributions to the field, including the isolation of the retroviral genome, the first analysis of the order of retroviral genes, and the discovery of the first retroviral cancer gene." (*IAV* p.396)

Duesberg reports that his scientific papers on AIDS "would constantly run into obstacles at every turn, from hostile peer reviews to reluctant editors."(*IAV* p.393) The rules mysteriously changed for "the *Proceedings of the National Academy of Sciences*, where Academy members such as Duesberg have an automatic right to publish papers without standard peer review." (*IAV* p.397) An editor rejected Duesberg's unique and provocative submission by bizarrely saying that it was not "original." And, supporting the case for the arbitrary make-it-up-as-you-go-along nature of abnormal AIDS science, a subsequent replacement editor decided tradition had to be completely ignored for this special case and the Duesberg paper had to be peer-reviewed because it was *"controversial."* (*IAV* p.397) It took several months of hostile reviewers negotiating with Duesberg before the paper was finally published. According to Duesberg, "Robert Gallo was asked to write a rebuttal, but never did." (*IAV* p.357) Strategic silent treatment is part of the arsenal of abnormal science.

The punishments for anyone standing up to totalitarian, abnormal science can be severe. Duesberg reports that "the AIDS establishment made its most effective counterattack by going after Duesberg's funding, the lifeblood of any scientist's laboratory. After coming out against the HIV theory, Duesberg was denied continuation of an N.I.H. Outstanding Grant by a group of scientists which included two who were proponents of the HIV paradigm and three scientists who never even reviewed the grant. When a review committee considered Duesberg's grant proposal a few months later, "they did . . . complain about Duesberg's questioning attitude as the major obstacle to funding him and singled out AIDS." (*IAV* p.402) Subsequently, "every one of his seventeen peer-reviewed grant applications to other federal state or private agencies—whether for AIDS research, on AZT and other drugs, or for cancer research—has been turned down." (*IAV* p.403) Thus did Duesberg come face to face with one of the telltale signs of abnormal and totalitarian science: blacklisting. The long arms of HIV/AIDS politics reached into his life at his university where "Several fellow professors" maneuvered "against Duesberg in various ways." His promotions in pay were "blocked" and he was denied "coveted graduate lecture courses." (*IAV* p.404)

One of the most dramatic and creepiest abnormal science moments in the Duesberg saga occurred in 1994 when a high-ranking geneticist from the N.I.H. flew to California to present Duesberg with an unpublished paper titled "HIV Causes AIDS: Koch's Postulates Fulfilled." Duesberg was asked to be a third author on a paper *he hadn't even collaborated on.* The paper had been commissioned by *Nature* editor and HIV theory proponent, John Maddox. Duesberg was warned by his high-ranking visitor that by continuing his opposition to the HIV theory he "would even risk his credentials for having discovered cancer genes." (*IAV* p.406) (The willingness to "disappear" the past is another one of the telltale signs of totalitarian science.) The geneticist told Duesberg that if he agreed to be an author on the paper it would "open the doors for Duesberg's reentry into the establishment." (*IAV* p 406) Duesberg said thanks but no thanks in the form of offering to write something for *Nature* that said the direct opposite of what that proposed unsigned paper posited.

A very thoughtful and philosophical man in many ways, Duesberg sought to understand the recalcitrant system that was making it so difficult for his ideas to be heard and tested, let alone prevail. He blamed it on "command science" which by his analysis, derived its power from three sources in the medical establishment: "(1) enforced consensus through peer review, (2) enforced consensus through commercialization and (3) the fear of disease, particularly infectious disease." (*IAV* p.452)

Because all serious medical scientists in America need grants from the NIH to survive, they often need to conform to the establishment viewpoint. While the "peer-review system" is supposed to be like an independent jury system, in reality, according to Duesberg, "a truly independent jury system would be fatal to the establishment." (*IAV* p.452) The result is "the peers serve the orthodoxy by serving their own vested interests." (*IAV* p.452) Duesberg warned that "as long as a scientist's work is reviewed only by competitors within his own field, peer review will crush genuine science." (*IAV* p.454)

Ominously for AIDS patients and the myriad victims of the real AIDS epidemic, Duesberg concluded that "Through peer review the federal government has attained a near-monopoly on science." (*IAV* p.454) Abnormal science loves the absolute power of monopolies. HIV became hegemonic because "a handful of federal agencies, primarily the NIH, dominate research policies and effectively dictate the official dogma . . . . By declaring the virus the cause of AIDS at a press conference sponsored by the Department of Health and Human Services, NIH researcher Robert Gallo swung the entire medical establishment and even the rest of the world, behind his hypothesis. Once such a definitive statement is made, the difficulty of retracting it only increases with time."(*IAV* p.454)

Duesberg criticized the huge conflict of interest in science that is caused by its commercialization. He argued that the FDA, by essentially banning competing therapies, often helps the pharmaceutical industry develop monopolies. Profits from products approved by the FDA often find their way back to scientists who sat in judgment on fellow scientists "in the form of patent royalties, consultantships, paid board positions, and stock ownership." (*IAV* p.455) In addition, "in order for a research product to find a market, the underlying hypothesis for the product must be accepted by a majority of the practitioners in the field." (*IAV* p.455) In the case of AIDS "commercial success can be achieved only by consensus. For example, an AIDS hypothesis would not be approved unless it miraculously cured AIDS overnight." (*IAV* p.455) Thus Gallo's royalties from an HIV patent as well as those with financial interest in HIV tests (Like William Haseltine and Max Essex) indicate that they may not be the most disinterested parties to make important decisions about the direction of AIDS research. And yet they were among the powerful inner circle of AIDS research. No wonder Duesberg often experienced forms of petulance and hostility from such characters rather than open-minded collegiality. In essence, by telling an inconvenient truth he was a threat to their lifestyles and reputations.

The third arm of the "command science" which Duesberg discusses goes in the opposite direction of the overriding conclusion of my newspaper's reporting about the real AIDS epidemic. Duesberg writes, "Traditionally, the power of medical science has been based on the fear of disease, particularly infectious disease. The HIV-AIDS establishment has exploited this instrument of power to its limit." (*IAV* p.456) Duesberg assumes that an infectious epidemic has essentially been invented out of whole cloth by incompetent epidemiology. His book would have been more accurately titled "Inventing the AIDS Epidemic." Duesberg accuses the CDC of delusional epidemiology driven by opportunism and hysteria. The manipulated paradigm of an infectious AIDS epidemic was used to create a "stampede," to create "irrational" fear in the public, to cynically manipulate, to mislead. And most importantly, from the Duesberg perspective, to build a lucrative new empire for the CDC.

While most of my work which began at *New York Native* supports the notion of a reign of intellectual dishonesty at the CDC, my conclusions about AIDS turn this part of the Duesbergian thesis on its head. Duesberg sees a devastating, apocalyptic epidemic being cynically and opportunistically *imagined*, and my reporting sees it as *existing—big time—and being concealed*. Other than HIV not being the cause of AIDS, the only thing Duesberg and I fundamentally agree on (in addition to the questionable behavior of many powerful individuals) is that the AIDS establishment was not really doing science as we expect it to be done. Duesberg might even agree with the premise that the science of AIDS was abnormal, totalitarian and even psychotic.

There is one other thing that Duesberg got right that deserves special mention. Duesberg performed an heroic whistle-blowing act during dark hours of the epidemic: his fearless adoption of a principled stand against the administration of AZT to AIDS patients. In a chapter of his book aptly titled, "With Therapies Like this, Who Needs Disease?", he discussed Azidothymidine, or AZT. About this very toxic drug that was being given to AIDS patients, Duesberg writes, "AZT kills dividing cells anywhere in the body—causing ulcerations and hemorrhaging; damage to hair follicles and skin; killing mitochondria, the energy cells of the brain; wasting away of muscles; and the destruction of the immune system and other cells. . . . Amazingly, AZT was first approved for treatment of AIDS in 1987 and then for prevention of AIDS in 1990." (*IAV* p.301) Duesberg didn't say it, but he didn't have to: AZT was more of a cruel, sadistic, toxic punishment than a medical treatment for AIDS patients.

AZT beautifully expressed the AIDS zeitgeist. AZT was invented in 1964 to kill cancer tumors, but the drug also effectively killed healthy growing tissues and was shelved without a patent because it was too toxic. Twenty years later scientists reported that it was capable of stopping HIV from replicating. Duesberg had serious doubts about even the basic AIDS research that was done with AZT which suggested that it could be given in small enough doses so that it would kill the virus without also killing the t-cells and other cells in the body. Not surprisingly, given the nature of AIDS science, the research that supported the safety of using AZT could not be subsequently replicated and showed that "the same low concentration [of AZT] that stops HIV also kills cells." (*IAV* p.313) Like much of the abnormal science of AIDS, if you looked diligently beneath one fraud, you could find yet another.

The person most responsible for foisting this quasi-genocidal toxic drug on AIDS patients was Sam Broder, the man who was Gallo's boss at the National Cancer Institute. He was the man responsible for the original questionable research suggesting that AZT could be given in doses that wouldn't harm patients. AIDS patients would pay a horrifying price for his scientific slovenliness. Duesberg notes, "Broder and his collaborators have never corrected their original reports, nor have they explained the huge discrepancies between their data and other reports." (*IAV* p.313)

Duesberg's critique of AZT gets even more devastating when he points out that the virus is dormant and therefore the virus "can only attack growing cells" and "like all other chemotherapeutic drugs, is unable to distinguish an HIV-infected cell from one that is uninfected. This has disastrous consequences on AZT-treated people; since only 1 in about 500 t-cells of HIV anti-body positive persons is ever infected, AZT must kill 499 good t-cells to kill just one that is infected by the hypothetical AIDS virus." (*LAV* p.313) In a sardonic understatement, Duesberg concluded, "It is a tragedy for people who already suffer from a t-cell deficiency." (*LAV* p.314) Needless to say, as time passes, giving people AZT sounds more and more unquestionably like a form of genocidal insanity or what I call "iatrogenocide." For a few who watched in horror as this transpired, it did *then*, too. Duesberg wrote "A toxic chemotherapy was about to be unleashed on AIDS victims, but no one had the time to think twice about its potential to destroy the immune systems of people who might otherwise survive." (*LAV* p.314) AZT belonged more in a court room as Exhibit A of a crimes against humanity trial than in the bodies of AIDS patients.

Unfortunately, given the all the surreal terror and hysteria of the time and the prevalent abject mentality of the patients, the gay community and its doctors wanted something—virtually anything—that could (or seemed to) address the problem. But make no mistake about it. There were also financial considerations that helped create the AZT disaster. Burroughs Welcome, the company that owned the patent on the drug, was eager to win approval for the treatment of AIDS by the FDA. Unfortunately for the AIDS patients, Burroughs Welcome's head researcher worked closely and effectively with Sam Broder to get FDA approval.

The process of testing the effectiveness of the drug was also highly questionable. The double blind, placebo-controlled studies of AZT on AIDS patients were not exactly double blind and placebo controlled. They were as abnormal as just about everything else in the Kafkaesque world of AIDS science. The list of things that went off the rails in the study was long. The study was stopped prematurely because the positive "results seemed stupendous." (*LAV* p.316) But as scientists looked more closely at the details of the study it turned out that the AZT trial was just as unreliable as much of the basic laboratory science that had launched AZT in the first place. More placebo patients had died than seemed reasonable. A close look at the study revealed that many of the AZT users had suffered horrific side effects which were downplayed even though they "more than abolished its presumed benefit." (*LAV* p.317)

When more information surfaced about the AZT trial, it turned out that the controls for the study were a complete mess. It was virtually impossible to conceal which patients were on AZT because in patients on AZT the drug killed bone marrow cells so quickly, that patients would come down with aplastic anemia, a not-hard-to-detect dreadful disease. According to Duesberg, "the patients, needless to say, often found out what they were taking" from clues like throwing up blood or changes in their blood counts. (*IAV* p.318) That had a grimly ironic effect on the study because those who discovered they were on the placebo, by comparing the tastes of their pills with the pills of those who were actually taking AZT, *wanted to take what they had been told was the life saving* AZT. It was a heartbreaking sign of the desperation and helplessness of their situation. According to Duesberg, "the patients had bought the early rumors of AZT's incredible healing powers, and they really did not want to take a placebo. Some of the placebo group secretly did use AZT, explaining the presence of its toxic side effects among those patients." (*IAV* p.318)

Because doctors easily noticed in the so-called "blinded" study that the AZT patients *seemed* to be doing better than the non-AZT patients, the study was ended early. The study's credibility was in shambles when it turned out that some of the patients on AZT had to be taken off of it because it was so toxic. According to Duesberg, "many of the patients simply could not tolerate AZT, and the physicians had to do something to save their lives." (*IAV* p.319) And "15 percent of the AZT group disappeared, possibly including patients with the most severe side effects." (*IAV* p.319) An inspection of documents pertaining to the study obtained under the Freedom of Information Act revealed a wide array of abnormalities in the study that suggested the study was one of the more notable frauds of the AIDS Era and Holocaust II.

While the initial results of the AZT study indicated an improvement of t-cells, it turned out that a temporary increase of t-cells did not really indicate that the patients were getting better. And there might have been some improvement of the patients from a broad spectrum antibiotic effect. The only problem was that *the drug was also toxically undermining the immune system*. It was opposite world science at its best. AZT was in essence becoming another cause of AIDS.

Tragically, even though the study was a scientific train wreck, the FDA approved AZT. The FDA panel that approved AZT included two paid consultants from Burroughs Wellcome. Duesberg notes, "the FDA endorsement could seem a cruel joke perpetrated by heartless AIDS scientists. Patients on AZT receive little more than white capsules surrounded by a blue band. But every time lab researchers order another batch for experimentation they receive a special label . . . A skull-and-crossbones symbol appears on background of bright orange, signifying an unusual chemical hazard." (*IAV* p.324)

Kary Mullis

The Nobelist with a Conscience

Kary Mullis is a biochemist who won the 1993 Nobel Prize for the Polymerase Chain Reaction. He, like Duesberg, was eventually troubled by the lack of evidence that HIV is the cause of AIDS. In the foreword he wrote for Duesberg's *Inventing the AIDS Virus*, he reported on the events that led to his criticism and ultimate confrontation with the AIDS establishment. Mullis had been hired by a firm called Specialty Labs to set up "analytic routines" for HIV. In the process of writing a report on the progress of his project, he went in search of support for this statement that was going to appear in the report: "HIV is the probable cause of AIDS." (*IAV* p.xi) He was puzzled that there was no paper to be found containing definitive proof of the statement and one that was "continually referenced in the scientific papers" about the epidemic. (*IAV* p.xi) He was puzzled that such a large enterprise involving so many scientists and growing numbers of sick and dying people did not rest on a solid foundation of a published paper that established with great certainty that HIV was the probable cause. A computer search came up with nothing. He started asking for the definitive reference at scientific meetings, but after attending ten or fifteen meetings over a period of a couple of years he "was getting pretty upset when no one could cite the reference." (*IAV* p.xi)

Mullis, without realizing it, had stumbled into the world of the abnormal totalitarian science of AIDS. He wrote, "I didn't like the ugly conclusion that was forming in my mind. The entire campaign against a disease increasingly regarded as a twentieth century Black Plague was based on a hypothesis whose origins no one could recall. That defied scientific and common sense." (*IAV* p.xii) It did however, make the opposite world kind of sense that is associated with abnormal science. Like the protagonist in Kafka's novel, Mullis had arrived at the Castle of HIV research. Science, logic, and common sense would be utterly beside the point. And pungent homodemiology (antigay epidemiology) was in the air, but Mullis, famous for his flamboyant, unapologetic heterosexuality, couldn't smell it.

When Mullis approached one of the founding fathers of the HIV/AIDS paradigm, the French discoverer of HIV himself, Luc Montagnier, he got the pass-the-buck, run-and-hide treatment that characterized the behavior of many of the top HIV authorities. When Mullis approached Montagnier at a San Diego scientific conference with his question Montagnier said, condescendingly, "Why don't you quote the report from the Centers for Disease Control?" (*IAV* p.xii) This from the future winner of a Nobel Prize for the discovery of HIV and one of the two people most responsible for an empire of HIV testing, stigmatization and toxic treatments that has entrapped millions of trusting people in its draconian public health agenda. When Mullis pointed out the weakness of the answer, that it didn't address the question, Montagnier suggested that Mullis look at the work on Simian Immunodeficiency Virus. Mullis responded that the research on that virus *didn't* remind him of AIDS at all, and didn't answer the more basic question about the whereabouts of "the original paper where somebody showed that HIV caused AIDS." (*IAV* p. xiii) At that point, Montagnier just abruptly walked away from Mullis. One could say that it was a typical interaction between the two different cultures of normal and abnormal science.

Mullis finally got his answer to the question when he happened to be listening to the radio in his car and heard an interview with Peter Duesberg. Mullis writes that Duesberg "explained exactly why I was having so much trouble finding the references that linked HIV to AIDS. *There weren't any.* No one had proved that HIV causes AIDS." (*IAV* p.xiii)

Interestingly, although Mullis is often considered a "Duesbergian," in the foreword to the Duesberg book, he writes, "I like and respect Peter Duesberg. I don't think he knows necessarily what causes AIDS; we have disagreements about that. But we're both certain about what *doesn't* cause AIDS." (*IAV* p.xiii)

Mullis also acknowledged in the foreword the outrageous iatrogenic tragedy that was occurring in the name of the HIV theory: "We have also not been able to discover why doctors prescribe a toxic drug called AZT (Zidovudine) to people who have no other complaint than the presence of antibodies to HIV in their blood. In fact, we cannot understand why humans would take that drug for any reason.' (*IAV* p.xiv)

Without formally calling HIV science anything like a totalitarian opposite world of abnormal science, he came very close when he wrote, "We cannot understand how all this madness came about, and having lived in Berkley, we've seen some strange things indeed. We know that to err is human, but the HIV/AIDS hypothesis is one hell of a mistake." (*IAV* p.xiv) It's fair to say that he seemed to sense that we were in a period of scientific psychosis.

When reporter Celia Farber asked Mullis about "the guardians of the HIV establishment, such as Gallo and [Anthony] Fauci," in a July, 1994 interview in *Spin* in July, 1994, Mullis said "I feel sorry for 'em" and "I want to have the story unveiled, but you know what? I'm just not the kick-'em-in-the-balls kind of guy. I'm a moral person, but I'm not a crusader. I think it's a terrible tragedy that it's happened. There are some terrible motivations of humans involved in this, and Gallo and Fauci have got to be some of the worst. . . . Personally, I want to see those fuckers pay for it a little bit. I want to see them lose their position. I want to see their goddamn children have to go to junior college. I mean who do we care about? Do we care about those people who are HIV-positive whose lives have been ruined? Those are the people I'm the most concerned about. Every night I think about this. I think, what is my interest in this? Why do I care? I don't know anybody dying of it. They're right about that, well except one of my girlfriend's brothers died of it, and I think he died of AZT."

In a chapter on AIDS in his own book, *Dancing Naked in the Mind Field*, Mullis angrily described the world of AIDS research: "In 1634 Galileo was sentenced to house arrest for the last eight years of his life for writing that the Earth is not the center of the universe but rather moves around the sun. Because he insisted that scientific statements should not be a matter of religious faith, he was accused of heresy. Years from now, people looking back at us will find our acceptance of the HIV theory of AIDS as silly as we find the leaders who excommunicated Galileo. Science as it is practiced today in the world is largely not science at all. What people call science is probably very similar to what was called science in 1634. Galileo was told to recant his beliefs or be excommunicated. People who refuse to accept the commandments of the AIDS establishment are basically told the same thing. 'If you don't accept what we say, you're out.'" (*DNITMF* p.180)

Mullis got the same kind of hostile and dismissive treatment from the scientific profession that Duesberg did: "The responses I received from my colleagues ranged from moderate acceptance to outright venom. When I was invited to speak about P.C.R. at the European Federation of Clinical Investigation in Toledo, Spain, I told them that I would like to speak about HIV and AIDS instead. I don't think they understood exactly what they were getting into when they agreed. Halfway through my speech, the president of the society cut me off. He suggested I answer some questions from the audience." (*DNITMF* p.181) Playing the all too predictable emotional blackmail card of AIDS orthodoxy, the president of the society then asked the first question himself—whether Mullis was being irresponsible and possibly causing people to not use condoms. The same game of AIDS emotional blackmail was played by virtually every institution of public health and science for three decades.

Unfortunately, in his book Mullis joined in the same kind of speculative, homodemiological free-for-all that many of the Duesbergians succumbed to, in which they concocted their own, usually heterosexist-flavored paradigms. Mullis's seat-of-the-pants paradigm was based on "highly mobile, promiscuous men sharing bodily fluids and fast lifestyles and drugs." (*DNITMF* p.182) Mullis accepted the basics of the CDC's deficient epidemiology without asking whether that too was more like the science of 1634. His encounter with abnormal science never got him close to lifting the veil on Holocaust II and the HHV-6 spectrum catastrophe and the viral and epidemiological passageways between AIDS, CFS, autism etc. But his challenge to the orthodoxy was certainly better than nothing and his notoriety got his views broadcast widely. Even *The New York Times* was forced to deal with Mullis, which they did in the characteristic arrogant and dismissive way that they dealt with all important challenges to the HIV hegemony. History will hopefully honor Mullis for using the leverage of his Nobel Prize for a humanitarian purpose.

Without trying to be, Mullis was briefly one of the more articulate voices of what could be called "the sorrow and the pity of Holocaust II." In his book, like Duesberg, he protested the use of AZT on AIDS patients. Mullis wrote, "About half a million people went for it. No one has been cured. Most of them are dead." (*DNITMF* p.185) And ne notes, "I was thinking that this technique of killing people with a drug that was going to kill them in a way hardly distinguishable from the disease they were dying from, just faster, was really out there on the edge of the frontier of medicine. (*DNITMF* p.186) It was also, unbeknownst to Mullis, on the frontier of homodemiological (and ultimately racist) medicine.

Robert Root-Bernstein

The Critical Genius

One of the most celebrated intellectuals who joined Duesberg and Mullis in their skepticism about the HIV theory of AIDS was Robert Root-Bernstein. Duesberg described him in *Inventing the AIDS Virus*: "Barely out of graduate school with a degree in the history of science, Root-Bernstein was awarded the MacArthur Prize fellowship—a five-year "genius grant— in 1981. This afforded him the opportunity to work alongside polio vaccine pioneer Jonas Salk, followed by a professorship at Michigan State University in physiology." (IAV p.245) Because of his background in the history of science, Root-Bernstein brought an academically analytical and philosophical perspective to the problems with the HIV theory. His book outlining his doubts about HIV, *Rethinking AIDS*, was published in 1993.

According to Duesberg, sometime in "early 1989 he had begun corresponding with Duesberg and other critics of the HIV hypothesis. Scouring the scientific literature, Root-Bernstein found hundreds of cases of AIDS-like diseases dating back throughout the twentieth century. These data he extracted into a letter published in *The Lancet* in April 1990, showing that Kaposi's sarcoma had not been as rare as supposed before the 1980s. The next month he fired off in rapid succession several more papers on the history of other AIDS diseases, all of which the same journal now rejected." (*IAV* p. 246) (*The Lancet*, especially under the guidance of Richard Horton, would play a major role in the maintenance of the HIV/AIDS paradigm throughout Holocaust II.)

In what Duesberg calls Root-Bernstein's major 1990 paper, "Do We Know the Cause(s) of AIDS?" he posited that "It is worth taking a skeptical look at the HIV theory. We cannot afford—literally, in terms of human lives, research dollars, and manpower investment—to be wrong. The premature closure leaves us open to the risk of making a colossal blunder." (*IAV* p. 246) Oh, yes we could.

Root-Bernstein's own book was not as Duesbergian as Duesberg probably would have liked because *he found a place for HIV in AIDS* by theorizing that it might be a part of some sort of multifactorial assault on the immune system that resulted in an autoimmune process. Duesberg had no patience with the autoimmune theories of AIDS for a number of reasons, including that fact that "if AIDS did result from autoimmunity, it would have spread out in its original risk group into the general population years ago, rather than striking men nine times out of ten. (*IAV* p.248)

Regardless of the fact that, like Duesberg, Root-Bernstein seems blissfully unaware of the presence of the heterosexism in the manner in which the ground-zero definition of AIDS was cooked up and despite his blind spot towards the existence of the chronic fatigue syndrome epidemic which resulted from the CDC habit of cherry-picking data, Root-Bernstein's book was a strong scientific wake-up call that urged a greater due diligence about the logic of AIDS and the emerging anomalous data that contradicted and challenged the prevailing paradigm. Root-Bernstein brought a distinctly Kuhnian sense of the nature of scientific process to his critique of HIV/AIDS and he seemed to be very aware (without exactly naming it) that it was engendering a culture of abnormal or totalitarian science. The epigrams in his books are like shots across the bow of the conventional view of AIDS. He quotes John Stuart Mill: "The fatal tendency of mankind to leave off thinking about a thing which is no longer doubtful is the cause of half their error." And Rollo May: "People who claim to be *absolutely* convinced that their stand is the only right one are dangerous. Such conviction is the essence not only of dogmatism but of its most destructive cousin, fanaticism. It blocks off the user from learning new truth and it is a dead giveaway of unconscious doubt." His quote from William Trotter M.D. may be been even more appropriate for a book on AIDS than even Root-Bernstein realized: "When we find ourselves entertaining an opinion about which there is a feeling that even to enquire into it would be absurd, unnecessary, undesirable, or wicked—we may know that the opinion is a nonrational one." (All quotes are from the frontispiece of *Rethinking AIDS*)

Root-Bernstein subsequently backed away from his position challenging HIV, but his book is so powerfully written that the damage it did to the credibility of the HIV paradigm could not be undone. Without flinching, in the preface he seems to have detected the bizarre nature of AIDS research: "I have read the medical literature assiduously, looking for studies that test our current theory of AIDS. I have analyzed and synthesized this information and found that our theory of AIDS is full of glaring holes, confusing contradictions, and outright discrepancies. I am saying nothing more than what the medical literature itself says about

AIDS. The only difference is that I am willing to say this in public, whereas most practitioners are not. (*RA* p.xiii) (The bit about the practitioners deserves a little attention from future historians of the epidemic. What does that tell us about the character and ethics of the people who did the hands-on management of AIDS patients?)

Root-Bernstein says that he wants to identify "the extent and nature of our ignorance" and that by doing so "we will be able to do something about it. In science, to define the problem correctly takes one more than halfway to its solution." (*RA* p.xiii) Very Kuhnian of him, but Root-Bernstein's biggest mistake may be that he was prepared to take the research he was studying at face value. With overabundance of optimism about science and scientists, he writes, "my critique of AIDS theory assumes that most of the published experiments and clinical observations are accurate" having been conducted by "many dedicated and hard-working scientists." (*RA* p.xii) That generous trust kind of contradicts the radical statement he makes near the end of the book: "I have put my scientific reputation on the line in this book in order to make certain that we accept nothing about AIDS uncritically." (*RA* p.373) Well, not exactly "nothing," if one assumes all "the published experiments and clinical observations are accurate." Therein lies the rub.

Root-Bernstein is basically saying that, *even giving* the basic researchers and their "facts" the benefit of the doubt, the interpretations and theories about the facts just don't compute. He begins his critical journey by pointing out that facts require theories and are not facts until they are "interpreted in light of a theory." (*RA* p.xiv) Where the "facts" about AIDS are concerned he notes that "the data are all easily validated by repeated observations and measurements, and yet may still be misunderstood. A great deal of evidence suggests, for example that we have attributed much too much to HIV . . . and too little to other causative agents." (*RA* p.xiv) He concluded that "it is imperative to rethink and research AIDS." (*RA* p.xv)

Like Thomas Kuhn, Root-Bernstein seems inadvertently to be conveying an image of science with more of a sinister potential than he realizes. He points out that "Most scientists believe that we understand AIDS and have trumpeted their belief to each other and the public as well . . . . This is the public face of AIDS—the face that is meant to exude confidence, to reassure." (*RA* p.1) But if this public face was false it makes one wonder to what degree the whole AIDS effort was an episode of misbegotten groupthink from the very beginning. He points out, "Scientists are much more reticent about revealing their other face—the one that displays their ignorance, confusion, and puzzlement over the aspects of the disease that they do not understand. The best kept secrets about AIDS are the questions unanswered, the puzzles unsolved, the contradictions unrecognized, and the paradoxes unformulated." (*RA* p.1) One doesn't know whether to laugh or cry over the casual way Root-Bernstein is basically telling us that the powerful AIDS establishment, almost a decade into the epidemic, was keeping two sets of books—an essential ingredient of abnormal science and homodemiology. Once again, like Kuhn, he may have been telling us far more about the real nature of science than he realized.

By calling his first chapter, "Anomalies," Root-Bernstein is signaling a belief in the power of unexpected findings and contradictions to force a critical reconsideration of paradigms, a distinctly Kuhnian notion of the way the process of normal science and scientific revolutions work, or are supposed to work. By doing so he is also in a way reassuring us that he was operating in a world of normal science which turned out—without him recognizing it—not to be the case at all. He asserts, "the existence of significant anomalies or departures from the regular expectations of the current theory must raise a red flag warning that our understanding of AIDS is not as profound as we might wish." (*RA*. p.1) Like any scientist in the collegial, reasonable world of normal science, he thought that the anomalies "are important enough to warrant serious rethinking of the causes and nature of AIDS." (*RA* p.2) We should note that, like Duesberg and many of the Duesbergians, he was not going all the way and calling for a rethinking of the ground zero epidemiology and nosology of AIDS.

The first anomaly he deals with is the fact that "there were a large number of pre-1979 AIDS-like cases that have not been accounted for in our current theories of AIDS." (*RA* p.21) He asks, "If HIV is a new and necessary cause of AIDS, as most AIDS researchers argue, what was the cause of these pre-1979 AIDS-like cases? Are there causes of acquired immune suppression other than HIV that may explain AIDS?" (*RA* p.21)

Root-Bernstein's second major anomaly focused on his contention that "HIV is neither necessary nor sufficient to cause AIDS." (*RA* p.21) He notes that the prevailing notion was that "infection with HIV is supposed to cause destruction of a specific type of immune system cell known as the t-helper or T4 cell." (*RA* p.22) Like more than a few others he noted the odd manner in which the government stepped in and basically established by fiat that the retrovirus HIV (or HTLV-III as it was then called) was the cause of AIDS. He also notes the troubling fact that the government announcement about the retrovirus happened "even before Gallo's paper [on HTLV-III] had undergone peer review and publication." (*RA* p.24) He also points out that the announcement was followed by a commitment to HIV research that made AIDS research "virtually synonymous with HIV research." (*RA* p.24) In effect, *all other avenues of research were closed off* from financial assistance or intellectual support from the HIV-obsessed AIDS establishment.

One curious and important point that Root-Bernstein acknowledges and historians won't want to let go of in reconstructions of that period is the fact that subsequently Gallo's so-called French co-discoverer, Luc Montagnier, had surprisingly indicated that HIV was actually *not sufficient* to cause AIDS. Montagnier had uncovered evidence that bacteria called mycoplasmas are necessary to stimulate HIV, making mycoplasmas at least a co-factor of AIDS, and possibly even more important than HIV, raising *the scandalous question of whether HIV was even the cause of AIDS.* Root-Bernstein also notes that, ironically, Gallo eventually also discovered his own co-factor, Human Herpes Virus Six (HHV-6) in AIDS patients, also potentially pulling the rug out from under Gallo's own HIV-alone-causes-AIDS theory. (*RA* p.26) The two so-called discoverers of the cause of AIDS laid the groundwork for their own eventual scientific fall from grace.

It's a tragedy for all the ultimate victims of HHV-6 and its family of viruses that Root-Bernstein didn't look harder at the virus. He might have helped make the public aware of the blossoming HHV-6 pandemic. He did recognize the chicken-or-egg threat that cofactors posed to the credibility of the HIV theory: "The only problem with the scenario is that it raises the question of which came first—the HIV or the cofactor." (*RA* p.26) Like a number of HIV critics, Root-Bernstein recounts the shocking paradigm-challenging moment at the 1992 International AIDS Conference at which it was announced *that there were AIDS patients without detectable HIV*: "Suddenly AIDS without HIV became big news because too many cases had surfaced to be ignored. There is no longer any doubt that HIV is not necessary to cause acquired immunodeficiency." (*RA*. p.29) Although at the time there were those who argued that there were not a large number of such cases, Root-Bernstein stood his ground, noting that "The actual number of HIV-negative AIDS cases is irrelevant. The existence of even a handful of HIV-negative AIDS cases is sufficient logically to raise doubts concerning the necessity of HIV as a cause of AIDS." (*RA* p.30)

Root-Bernstein came as close as he could to stumbling into the raw truth about the pandemic of HHV-6 when he hypothesized that one possibility implied by the HIV-negative cases was "that there is a second epidemic masquerading under the guises of AIDS, which has yet to have been detected and separated out from AIDS." (RA p.30) We now know that there *was* that other HIV-negative AIDS epidemic and it was, to the detriment of the health and human rights of all the patients involved, separated politically from the so-called AIDS epidemic. He was a witness to a growing state of medical apartheid that was concealing the HHV-6 catastrophe without realizing it.

His third anomaly focused on the mystery of where HIV was in the body and how it was transmitted. He pointed out that HIV was "anything but typical of sexually transmitted diseases. It can take hundreds of exposures for HIV for transmission to occur at all." (RA p. 31) It was rare to find HIV in semen. The way that HIV actually was transmitted was complex and didn't fit the STD picture the AIDS public health establishment was promoting—another strike against the consistency and trustworthiness of those guiding the AIDS effort. The data about HIV suggested "it is probable that those who become infected must be exposed repeatedly to many HIV carriers or have some unusual susceptibility for the virus." (RA p.38)

His fourth anomaly focused on the fact that people could be exposed to HIV without seroconverting. Given the numbers of sexual partners of HIV positives who did not seroconvert and oddities like the fact that prostitutes who did not use intravenous drugs rarely became HIV positive, he concluded, "HIV cannot be a sexually transmitted disease, in the usual sense of the term." (RA p.41) Other studies suggested that people had to be immune suppressed *before* they became HIV positive. He asserted, "Individuals with normal immune function should therefore be resistant to HIV." (RA p.42) And that comes very close to saying flat out that HIV is an effect rather than a cause.

As we have said, like most (but not all) of the heterosexuals in the Duesberg camp, he concluded that "one clear implication of these studies is that the non-drug abusing heterosexual community should have little or no risk of HIV or AIDS." (RA p.43) Root-Bernstein was blissfully unaware, like all the rest of the Duesbergians, that a highly variable epidemic of HHV-6 was raging all around him while being hidden epidemiologically behind the euphemism such as "chronic fatigue syndrome." Like most Duesbergians, his main agenda often appears to be debunking the myth of heterosexual AIDS.

Given that HHV-6 would ultimately be seen as a trigger for some cases of multiple sclerosis, it is interesting to note in passing that Root-Bernstein writes about one unlucky heterosexual woman who did seroconvert to HIV "suffered from multiple sclerosis, which had been repeatedly treated with immunosuppressive drugs." (RA p.44) Again in a French Farce moment of the tragic AIDS story, he may have been an unopened door away from the smoking gun.

The entire Duesberg camp seemed determined to provide themselves a margin of safety that separated them and their fellow heterosexuals from the possibility of the scarlet letter diagnosis of AIDS. Root-Bernstein gave his fellow heterosexual Duesbergians the ultimate reassurance when he wrote that "the transmission of HIV through heterosexual intercourse is so rare that two heterosexuals without identified risks for AIDS have an equal probability of being struck by lightning, dying in a commercial airplane crash, or developing AIDS." (RA p.44) Unfortunately, he could not provide the same reassurance for the heterosexual Duesbergians about chronic fatigue syndrome, autism or any of the other medical problems related to the unrecognized immune-system-challenging epidemic of HHV-6. The one that was hiding in plain sight.

One of the most damaging facts for the credibility of the HIV theory was the matter of transmission (or non-transmission) to health care workers. He writes that "there have however, been more than 6,000 verified cases of health care workers reporting subcutaneous exposure to HIV-infected blood or tissue as a result of needle-stick injuries, surgical cuts, broken glass and so forth. . . . And yet only a few dozen health care workers are known to have become HIV seropositive during the entire decade of the 1980s in the United States. (RA p.44) He was all too unaware that health care workers were, however, coming down with illnesses associated with the so-called AIDS cofactor, HHV-6, and being diagnosed with chronic fatigue syndrome and other diagnoses on the HHV-6 spectrum. Being in the health care field actually was one of the biggest risks for developing chronic fatigue syndrome. Root-Bernstein, again relying on the CDC's questionable ground zero epidemiology, notes that AIDS was not being transmitted to patients by health care workers. (The same could not necessarily be said for HHV-6 and chronic fatigue syndrome.) He accuses the HIV establishment of not being sufficiently skeptical but the truth is that his own skepticism never really went deep enough. But in his favor there is the undeniable fact that he did ask the kind of provocative questions that *should* have helped alert the scientific profession that something *was* terribly amiss in the world of AIDS research. The fact that most of his colleagues, throughout the three decades of Holocaust II, didn't listen to warnings like his and put their heads in the sand will be puzzled over by historians for a long time to come.

Root-Bernstein, on some level, was not-so-quietly outraged by what he was seeing and brought a much-needed dose of sarcasm to the field when he asked if "HIV is so radically different from all other viruses that we cannot compare it to them?" (*RA* p.42) Actually, he should have asked if there was something so radically different about the science and epidemiology of AIDS that no educated and decent person in their right mind could possibly understand it. He certainly seemed to be onto the fact that whatever the cause of AIDS was, *if it was a virus, it had to be unique.* Which is exactly what the multi-systemic virus HHV-6 turned out to be. If there is a virus more unique than HHV-6 I would like to know what it is.

Root-Bernstein's fifth anomaly concerned the ability of some people to fight off an infection of HIV. Some people never even developed antibodies to the retrovirus. Some tested negative for the virus years after testing positive. Some tested positive and remained perfectly healthy with intact immune systems. He caught a whiff of the Kafkaesque politics that controlled the developing AIDS empire (and its homodemiological reign of abnormal science) when he wrote, "Oddly, the ability of adults and infants to control or eliminate HIV infection in the absence of medical treatment is not seen by researchers as a source of hope for those at risk for AIDS but rather as a new public health threat." (*RA* p.54) In that lucid statement he inadvertently comes face to face with the looniness of HIV/AIDS "science" and kind of shrugs his shoulders in puzzlement.

Because Root-Bernstein, like nearly all the Duesbergians, didn't seem to grasp the sexual (and ultimately racist) politics driving the psychology of the establishment he was challenging, he didn't understand why his statement "that even people in high risk groups who may have initially had multiple contacts with HIV may successfully combat the viral infection" (*RA* p.54) would not comfort a heterosexist scientific establishment that was determined not to look back at its possible epidemiological and virological mistakes. No "source of hope" that didn't involve social control, stigmatization and the administration of toxic drugs could be given to gays (or blacks) in AIDS epidemiology and virology. The AIDS agenda was inexorable and unforgiving. Public health had adopted a scorched earth policy against those it was supposedly helping.

When Root-Bernstein brings up the evolving latency period of AIDS, he may have touched on the most important anomaly of all. He writes that "one of the oddest observations that strikes a historian of the epidemic is that the latency period—the estimated time lag between HIV infection and the development of clinical AIDS—has expanded almost yearly. In 1986, the figure was less than two years; in 1987, it was raised to three; in 1988, it became five; in 1989, ten; and as of the beginning of 1992, the latency period was calculated to be between ten and fifteen years (RA p.55) He wondered whether it was because the virus had become less virulent, or had killed people with the highest risk lifestyles—in terms of drugs and multiple sex partners—first. He concluded that "attributing AIDS to nothing more than an infection by HIV is too simplistic. It leaves too much unexplained and creates too many anomalies to be a satisfying scientific explanation. HIV is not sufficient to explain the anomalies of AIDS. These anomalies represent the challenge of understanding AIDS. A more thorough and skeptical analysis of the data is needed." (RA p.56) Blind to the heterosexism hardwired into the "science" and epidemiology he was confronting, he didn't understand that an anomaly-riddled HIV theory was a very adequate and politically useful scientific explanation in the opposite world of totalitarian, abnormal science that AIDS represented. Something far more politically and emotionally satisfying than reason and logic was at work here.

A rather democratic, collegial attitude about science and scientists comes across in Root-Bernstein's book. He was not one to put people he disagreed with on the rack. (One doubts that the HIVists would ever return the compliment.) He asserted optimistically, "anomalies, problems, paradoxes, and contradictions are only the incentives for research. If no one pays attention to them, they are fruitless. Even when they are identified and scrutinized, they are only a beginning; they define the areas of our ignorance." (RA. p.57) Unbeknownst to him, the gang he was dealing with was not interested in "our ignorance." They had a commitment to not paying attention to "anomalies, problems, paradoxes, and contradictions."

Having initially accepted the basic ground zero definition of AIDS with its subsequent ground zero epidemiology—a big mistake with horrific consequences—he is left praising HIV with faint damning: "The upshot of the discussion will be that HIV has not satisfied any established criteria for demonstrating disease causation. Thus, although, there is no doubt that HIV is an integral player in the drama of AIDS, we cannot say, for certain that it is beyond a doubt, a solo actor doing a monologue." (RA p.58)

Like others who concocted their own theories of AIDS causation before him, Root-Bernstein heads off into the wild goose chase of multifactorial causation where HIV has "a whole cast of supporting characters that foster its villainous work." (*RA* p.58)

Root-Bernstein does at least give *some* lip service to the importance of digging under the surface of the early epidemiology of AIDS in his chapter on the role of HIV in AIDS. He notes the disturbing history of the unstable definition of AIDS that always seemed to be changing. He was troubled by the notion that there were people in the high-risk group with AIDS indicator diseases like Kaposi's sarcoma *who were HIV-negative*. He noted that "AIDS, in short, has become a schizophrenic disease . . . Some people are AIDS patients if they develop opportunistic infections even in the absence of evidence of HIV, and in the presence of HIV, almost any rare disease is diagnostic for AIDS regardless of whether the person has other, more fundamental causes of immune suppression." (*RA* p.63) And, at the time his book was written in the early 90s, the CDC was proposing a change in the definition of AIDS that meant "People may be diagnosed as having AIDS even if they have no infections typical of AIDS, as long as they have a significantly low number of T-helper cells and antibody to HIV." (*RA* p.63) What Root-Bernstein had to say about the proposed change came into close proximity of *this book's thesis*: "The reason for this latest definitional alteration is social and economic, not scientific. AIDS activists are now dictating how AIDS is to be diagnosed and who is to be included in the count. For them, the issue is not one of correct diagnosis or elucidating the cause of AIDS; it is the understandable desire to increase access to health care." (*RA* p.64) And what great humanitarians those activists were, and what wonderful health care AZT and its toxic siblings turned out to be! What Root-Bernstein failed to perceive was that the definition of AIDS, drawn from the wrong first impressions of the real HHV-6 pandemic, was a groupthink-biased epidemiological product developed by scientists who looked at the epidemic through heterosexist and retroviral glasses.

Those who define the terms of an epidemic can control how large or small it appears at any point, which gives them de facto political power not only over the epidemic but potentially—with the broad and invasive powers of public health sanctions—a whole country. The chief definers would also be the chief deciders of the AIDS public health agenda. One of the great ironies of Root-Bernstein's often cogent criticisms of AIDS is that he understands the political nature of this phenomena but comes to a conclusion about the politics of the AIDS epidemic which is actually the direct opposite of the inconvenient truth. And it is tragically typical of most of the Duesbergians. Root-Bernstein points out that the CDC could say that AIDS cases doubled by just changing the definition, or what he called "definitional fiat." (RA p.64) He is on the money that the epidemiological appearance of AIDS was controlled by "definitional fiat" but not in the statistically upward direction he and the Duesbergians imagined. In truth, it was the CDC's heterosexist and ultimately racist "definitional fiat" that was keeping the public from seeing the connection of AIDS and CFS (and ultimately autism) in an exponentially larger unified multisystemic epidemic via the pathogen HHV-6. The difference between Root-Bernstein vision of the epidemic and the truth was the difference between using public relations to overstate an epidemic and using public relations to conceal one

Like the point in a movie when the audience sees a protagonist come within inches of a culprit without the protagonist realizing it, Root-Bernstein came tantalizingly close to the truth about the HHV-6 catastrophe when he notes, "We must be absolutely certain that HIV is not an epiphenomenon of AIDS before we assert that it is a primary cause. The fact that it is an extremely frequent finding in AIDS patients is not logically compelling. It is only suggestive. Other active infections, such as cytomegalovirus, are nearly universal among AIDS patients. If both are correlated with AIDS, which is the cause?" (RA p.66) He was *so very close* to the real issue of HHV-6 at that point and yet ultimately so far away.

He zeroed in on the tragic truth about HIV when he wrote, "HIV may be an epiphenomenon of immune suppression rather than a necessary cause."(RA p.66) This very bright history-aware thinker was also on the money when he wrote "one gaping lacuna in the AIDS definition" was that "There are no criteria listed in any definition of AIDS that allowed for a person to fight off AIDS or to be cured of it." (RA p.67) He noted that such a definition was "a medical novelty." (RA p.67) Actually, the whole field of AIDS research was one big cockamamie medical novelty. He thoughtfully notes that "this makes AIDS the first disease that no one can survive, by definition. Not only is this description of AIDS logically bankrupt, it sends the demoralizing and inaccurate message to people with HIV or AIDS that they have a disease that is not worth fighting." (RA p.68) Such a logically bankrupt demoralizing definition is of course, the work of the abnormal science of homodemiology on a productive day. But how could Root-Bernstein know that something like homodemiology was in play if it was a construct completely absent from his conceptual universe?

Like Thomas Kuhn, Root-Bernstein seems keenly aware that the psychology of scientists affects the decision-making process. In frustration, he asks questions like "Why is it so difficult for them to admit . . . that AIDS may have more than one cause?" (*RA* p.84) He knows he is dealing with "dogma" but he doesn't consider the possibility that the confounding issues like the threat to institutional pride and credibility as well as serious potential financial losses would follow upon the admission that HIV was not the one and only cause of AIDS. Those pedestrian kinds of conflict of interest could have done the trick even if the more esoteric underlying issues of heterosexism and racism were not involved. But, unfortunately, *they were.*

Again, Root-Bernstein asserted the point that most of the other Duesbergians believed as an article of faith about the risk of AIDS to heterosexuals: "If AIDS is a simple, sexually transmitted virus then it should be running rampant in the heterosexual community by now." (*RA* p.87) Cut to the real epidemic: HIV may have not been running rampant in the heterosexual community, but HHV-6 (and its spectrum of related viruses) certainly was and if the Duesbergians could have just looked behind the euphemism of "chronic fatigue syndrome," they would have had a ring side seat from which to watch the real heterosexual epidemic of variable immune dysfunction unfold all around them.

Root-Bernstein insists, "Evidence of the necessity of co-factors for HIV was found at the outset. (*RA* p.92). What he didn't realize is that co-factors were a political and economic threat to those seeking Nobel prizes for HIV and those members of the public health (and pharmaceutical) establishment who were rolling out a draconian heterosexist (and eventually racist) toxic agenda around the seeming inexorable public health logic of HIV control. One can't assign medical Pink Triangles based on a salad bar of co-factors.

Like the brightest Duesbergians, Root-Bernstein notes that an unprecedented scientific logic was afoot, one that cavalierly discarded Koch's postulates. He describes the issue succinctly when he writes "The logic of Koch's postulates is straight forward: Demonstrate that one, and only one, organism is associated both with the occurrence of a specific disease and with its onset by isolating and controlling its transmission independent of other factors." (*RA* p.95) He emphasizes that "Every controllable infectious disease known to medical science . . . has been solved by following Koch's postulates." (*RA* p.95) The totalitarian, Kafkaesque quality of AIDS research is inadvertently but beautifully captured in Root-Bernstein's statement that "the fact that HIV does not satisfy Koch's postulates does not convince HIV proponents that it is not the cause of AIDS. On the contrary, 'knowing' that HIV causes AIDS most researchers reject Koch's postulates." (RA p.99) The mad hatters of AIDS research generally hated to be confused by the facts or standards of proof and logic. Root-Bernstein underlines the outrageousness of this new form of "scientific reasoning" when he writes, "AIDS researchers have ignored previous criteria for establishing disease causation in favor of ad hoc inventions of their own." (RA p.100) Ad hoc inventions by AIDS researchers? Hello!

Root-Bernstein points out how flimsy the original evidence for HIV was: "What is somewhat astonishing is that in 1984, when Gallo first championed HIV as the cause of AIDS, the correlation between HIV and AIDS was not even particularly convincing." (RA p.101) (It was somewhat astonishing *if* you didn't know how HIV charlatan Robert Gallo and his homies rolled.)

Gymnastic attempts were made by scientists to concoct criteria to replace Koch's postulates in such a way that they could be conveniently used to prove HIV was the cause of AIDS. You could say that gays were such very special people that the HIV/AIDS scientists wanted to come up with very special rules that a proved that this very special virus was infecting *them* in a very special way, and mostly *only them*. In a Procrustean manner, the rules would be shaped in a heterosexist, racist, and illogical manner to fit the evidence and support a pre-ordained biased conclusion. This is how abnormal science and homodemiology seized the day.

Root-Bernstein sums up the infernal game being played in this scientific madhouse: "In short, HIV does not satisfy any of the etiological criteria that existed prior to its discovery, and the etiological criteria that have been developed since are all logically flawed." (RA p.103) Calling this kind of science abnormal or psychotic almost seems like an understatement.

In a rather gentlemanly tone Root-Bernstein *does indict* a whole generation of doctors and scientists who stood by as collaborators, enablers and useful idiots of this scientific debacle when he writes, "Given this state of affairs, attempts to modify Koch's postulates after the assertion that the causative agent has been identified smack of a posteriori reasoning. Such reasoning is always suspect to logicians and should be equally suspect to physicians and scientists as well." (RA p.104). In the world of normal science maybe, but not in the heterosexist world of abnormal science and homodemiology.

Knowing that scientific change only occurs when a new paradigm is offered that is more logical and attractive than the prevailing one, Root-Bernstein takes his own out for a spin. He plays around with the notion that AIDS may be "a synergistic or stepwise multifactor disease." (RA p.108) He tosses into his speculative multifactor salad of immunosuppressive elements: things like semen and addictive or recreational drugs. He spends much of the rest of his book backing up his contention that "there is a well-established set of diseases that have many of the characteristics of AIDS—multiple disease causing-agents—that may provide an as yet untested model for AIDS." (RA p.109) One thing that strikes one as refreshing about Root-Bernstein throughout his book is that, unlike many of the people in the Duesberg camp, he doesn't seem to be faithfully married to his own dogma. In the spirit of keeping an open mind, he asserted, "The case that HIV causes AIDS is still open, and surprises are still possible." (RA p.109) By exploring a number of possible non-infectious causes of immunosuppression like semen, recreational drugs, anesthesia, surgery, pharmaceutical agents like antibiotics, blood transfusions, clotting factors, and aging itself, he tries to build a case that any combination of these factors might lead to immunosuppression and that the assumption that HIV "is the only immunosuppressive agent in those at risk for AIDS and the only agent necessary to explain the immune suppression that characterizes the syndrome." (RA p.111) He was saying that many different combinations of elements might be creating a perfect immunological storm.

He also explored the possibility that AIDS was the result of multiple, concurrent infections, arguing, with a somewhat overzealous heterosexist bias, that "Perhaps no other group in history has ever sustained anything like the disease overload experienced by highly promiscuous homosexual men and intravenous drug abusers, with the sole exception of people who live in Third World nations. . ." (RA p.149) While he explores a laundry list of infections that he thinks may synergize into AIDS (CMV, EBV, HBV, mycoplasma and others), he once again comes painfully close to the smoking gun of the HHV-6 catastrophe at the core of Holocaust II when he writes about HHV-6 that it "may be of particular importance in AIDS because Robert Gallo's laboratory has demonstrated that it is common among people at risk for AIDS and acts as a cofactor to increase infectivity and cell-killing by HIV under test tube conditions." (RA p.152) (Not to mention that it was also found in HIV-negative patients with the heterosexual not-so-distant cousin of AIDS—chronic fatigue syndrome—but that was something he seemed destined to not know *anything* about.)

Root-Bernstein devotes an interesting chapter to the notion that AIDS may be a disease of autoimmunity noting, "autoimmunity has a wide range of manifestations in AIDS patients and people at risk for AIDS." (*RA* p.185) He argued that "autoimmunity directed at lymphocytes is only one of the many forms of autoimmunity that manifest themselves during the process of AIDS." (*RA* p.190) He certainly had a much more complex vision of what was going on in AIDS than the rather simplistic (and manufactured) HIV-infecting T-4 cell disease image that the patients and the public were indoctrinated with. When historians go back and try to determine why scientists and epidemiologists didn't recognize that AIDS and chronic fatigue syndrome actually were part of the same variable but unified epidemic, they will wonder why Root-Bernstein's description of the complexities of AIDS didn't have an eye-opening impact on anyone who was watching the emergence of chronic fatigue syndrome in the general population at that point in the late 80s and early 90s. The honest, open-minded critics of the HIV theory of AIDS and those concerned about CFS were just ships passing in the night. (And the passengers on those ships were replete with white heterosexual privilege.)

Root-Bernstein wrote, "Many AIDS patients develop an autoimmune form of arthritis; autoantibodies directed at muscle proteins; and symptoms similar to both Sjögren's syndrome and systemic lupus erythematosus, including skin rashes, kidney damage, and antibodies against DNA, thyroglobulin, and adrenocorticosteroids." (*RA* p.191) He was not ready to just glibly attribute all these complications to HIV. The patients back then would have probably been better served if the people attending to their health hadn't been forced by the establishment to adopt the simplistic "HIV-only" and "T-4 cells-mainly" way of looking at the disease

Root-Bernstein was concerned that "HIV is only one of a multitudinous cast that cooperate to produce autoimmunity." (*RA* p.203) He felt that scientists were making a major mistake in ignoring "the huge number of other infectious agents that are also present in AIDS patients, often concurrently." (*RA* p.203) Among those concurrent infections was of course, one very special one, the star of the multisystemic biomedical catastrophe, being mostly ignored and hiding behind the alibi that it was just another not-so-interesting infection that AIDS patients supposedly got secondarily: HHV-6.

Root-Bernstein was particularly interested in CMV which was a major viral problem in AIDS and which he thought could cause autoimmunity when it combined with other infections. He was especially intrigued by the possibility that CMV or some other herpes virus (he didn't bring up the then recently discovered HHV-6 here) was causing encephalitis or demyelization in a significant number of AIDS patients. The AIDS establishment of course, was determined to blame this, like everything else in AIDS, on HIV alone, to which he replied, "My opinion is that we have asked HIV to be responsible for too much of AIDS." (*RA* p.209) This statement from Root- Bernstein captures how potentially damaging this over-simplification of AIDS into "HIV T-4 cell disease" was: ". . . autoimmunity has many manifestations in AIDS besides that directed at lymphocytes. The causes of lymphocyte depletion may be entirely unrelated to causes of specific autoimmune symptoms, such as demyelization and thrombocytopenia, that are frequent concomitants of AIDS. It is possible that HIV may play the major role in one form of autoimmunity, and none in others. A concerted effort is needed to disentangle the many different forms of autoimmunity. As these various manifestations become distinct, they will inevitably call for new treatments unrelated to retroviruses." (*RA* p.218) Unfortunately, Root-Bernstein didn't realize just how much control the HIV mafia would continue to have for decades over the AIDS public health agenda—control that AIDS patients would pay an unprecedented medical and social price for. And they would hardly be alone.

Root-Bernstein seems to have been operating under the belief that the genteel Thomas Kuhn universe of normal science was the one he was living in when he wrote, "The purpose of theorizing is to cause us to rethink things we thought we understood in order to go out and ask new questions." (*RA* p.219) To which the AIDS establishment snarkily could probably have replied, "And who said anything about asking questions?" Given the relationship of AIDS to chronic fatigue syndrome and all the other manifestations of HHV-6 it is quite ironic to hear Root-Bernstein state ever so innocently and plaintively, "There may be major discoveries still left to be made not only concerning AIDS but the entire field of immunology—discoveries that may illuminate many diseases besides AIDS. With these discoveries will come new possibilities for treatment." (*RA* p.219) Unfortunately, in the nasty Realpolitik of Holocaust II, it was simply not meant to be.

As we have pointed out, the whole Duesbergian critical-thinking and re-thinking movement seemed to revolve around attempts to prove that heterosexuals were essentially *not at risk* for what the CDC called AIDS. They were on thin ice because they depended upon the CDC's ground zero epidemiological judgment calls. In a chapter titled "Who is at Risk for

AIDS and Why," Root-Bernstein throws down the gauntlet: "If exposure to HIV is sufficient to cause AIDS, then everyone should be at equal risk, and AIDS should develop at an equal rate among different risk groups once infection has become established. Clearly that is not the case." (*RA* p.220) Earth to Root-Bernstein: HHV-6 and chronic fatigue syndrome. For starters.

Root-Bernstein, like all the rest of the Duesbergians, confused the threat of AIDS with the threat of being diagnosed HIV positive. Just because heterosexuals were not being labeled as HIV-positive or as having AIDS, didn't mean that a large number of heterosexual Americans were not starting to develop a broad range of immunological dysfunctions and other problems that resembled the AIDS spectrum of pathologies. The Duesbergians, keenly unaware of the wildfire of HHV-6 and CFS, loved to make statements similar to Root-Bernstein's that "Some calculations place the figure of contracting AIDS from a heterosexual without risk factors as low as 2 in 1 million or the same risk as being struck by lightning." (*RA* p.220) About as close to never as you can get.

Working with the CDC's flawed, heterosexist data on what was AIDS and what wasn't, Root-Bernstein goes to town on the gay community and writes, "Until we understand exactly what these predisposing factors are for each separate risk group, we will not be able to identify, treat, control, or eliminate the risks of AIDS." (*RA* p.222) Never in the history of mankind has there been such a showboating of intense benevolent interest in understanding the gay community, and with understanding like this the gay community didn't need enemies. As could be predicted by this heterosexual noblesse-oblige-driven journey into the sex and drug habits of the gay community, the blame for AIDS is laid (more or less) on "promiscuous, drug-abusing, multiple-infected gay men." (*RA* p.232) You know, people who like to party. Coincidentally, since the general heterosexual population was not "promiscuous, drug-abusing, multiple-infected," they had no worry about contracting what the CDC had branded as "AIDS." Unless, of course—and this was not on Root-Bernstein's radar—they came in contact with the immune-system-compromising buzz-killer of a casually transmitted virus, HHV-6.

While Root-Bernstein also points to the multiple-infection lifestyle of drug users and the multiple-immunosuppressive risks of transfusion patients and hemophiliacs—and some infants born to parents with immunosuppressive drug-using lifestyles—they do little to take away from the notion that the driving force of his theorizing about AIDS was the same kind of GRID-think, or Got-AIDS-Yet?-think, that dominated the AIDS establishment's ground zero epidemiology. GRID-think was the heterosexist gift that just kept on giving for three decades. Root-Bernstein looked at AIDS as the inexorable price that some gays paid for an overindulgent lifestyle. That kind of thinking, which made heterosexuals feel comfy-cozy inside the Schadenfreude of their invulnerable biomedical cocoon, blinded society to the catastrophe of CFS, autism and everything else on the HHV-6 spectrum.

While the critical mission in his chapter on immunosuppression in AIDS was to expose the power of co-factors in the so-called AIDS risk groups, he may have inadvertently discovered that a broader definition of AIDS that focused on a wide range of indicators of immunosuppression (or more appropriately, immune dysfunction) would have shown that there was a far bigger and more variable AIDS or AIDS-like epidemic happening *even in the gay community itself.* In his chapter on the matter he promises to "show . . . that significant immune suppression is present in large numbers of people in high-risk groups for AIDS in the *absence* of HIV infections. Sometimes the degree of immune suppression is equal to, or even greater than, that experienced by HIV-positive, matched patients." (*RA* p.259) In the world of normal science this should have been all you needed to know to have an anomaly-driven epiphany that HIV was probably *not* the cause of AIDS. But not in the opposite world of abnormal science that Root-Bernstein was unknowingly adrift in. If that wasn't enough, he points out that "many people in the high-risk groups for AIDS have significant immune impairment prior to contracting an HIV infection and are thus susceptible to both infection and the effects of infection than are immunologically healthy individuals." (*RA.* p.259) It's almost like he's saying that people have HIV-negative AIDS (something CFS turned out to be) before they have HIV-positive AIDS. He strengthened his case by noting that "it is clear that acquired immune deficiencies do not require the presence of HIV infection." (*RA.* p.259) The chronic fatigue syndrome epidemic that he, for whatever reason, didn't know about was certainly a neon sign for *that* notion.

Rather than suggest that there may be some other agent responsible for both HIV-positive AIDS and what looked like HIV-negative AIDS in the gay community, (while also not considering that there might be an unseen HIV-negative immunological event going on in the general population— which there was), he instead went on a fishing expedition for *infections associated with gays* that could support a multi-factorial HIV-plus-something-else theory of AIDS. It's a shame that he didn't take the HIV-negative AIDS issue and run with it, launching an all-out assault on the HIV theory. As they say, he who would wound the lion must kill him. He was merely wounding the paradigm. If HIV-negative AIDS was nature's way of saying flat out that HIV couldn't be the cause of AIDS, then Root-Bernstein wasn't listening closely enough. It's amazing that Root-Bernstein didn't see more red flags considering that he wrote, "In fact, a large body of evidence demonstrates that significant immune suppression occurs in the absence of HIV infection in groups at high risk for AIDS but not among low-risk groups. HIV seropositive individuals within each identified risk group are no more immune suppressed than those who are HIV seronegative, as long as they do not contract other active infections." (RA p.261) He also reports that "the laboratories of Jerome Groopman and Robert Gallo [of all people] found that as many as 50 to 80 percent of HIV-seronegative homosexual men and hemophiliacs had significantly reduced T-helper/T-suppressor ratios during 1984." (RA p.262) Again, it was as though they had found a big gay HIV-negative epidemic of immunosuppression that might have pulled the rug out from under the HIV-positive paradigm that was about to trap the gay community in the draconian and toxic public health agenda I call Holocaust II.

While Root-Bernstein points to studies that suggest that Cytomegalovirus (CMV), the under-appreciated virus that the CDC initially suspected was the cause of AIDS, was responsible for the immunosuppression in HIV-negative men who were immune-suppressed, it was the HIV-negativity itself rather than the CMV that should have sent everyone back to the nosological and epidemiological drawing board to see if they had overlooked some other new infection—like the recently (at that point) discovered HHV-6. It was a huge missed opportunity, to say the least.

One of the most damning studies for the HIV theory of AIDS "consisted of an immunological and infectious disease evaluation of 100 'healthy' homosexual men in Trinidad in 1987 carried out by Robert Gallo, William Blattner, and their colleagues. Nearly all the men in the study, whether they were HIV seropositive or not, had a significant depletion of T-helper cells." (RA p.265) On top of that they also discovered "that some HIV-infected men had normal T-helper cells. Thus, HIV alone did not uniquely signify concomitant immune suppression." (RA p.265) Once again, that might have finished HIV off if research was occurring in the world of normal science rather than in one guided by homodemiology.

Given the confusion between CMV and HHV-6 in AIDS, Root-Bernstein again came close to peering into the HHV-6 catastrophe when he wrote, "In fact, although very few studies have been performed, cytomegalovirus appears to be as good a marker for increasing immune incompetence as HIV. R.J. Biggar and his colleagues reported in 1983 (prior to the isolation of HIV) that a very good correlation existed between the excretion of CMV in the semen of homosexual men and the degree of the immune suppression." (*RA*. p.279) CMV was good. But the HHV-6 family, as it turns out, was better.

And similarly, given the role of EBV in CFS (sometimes considered to be HIV-negative AIDS), which some people had called "chronic mono" because of the EBV reactivation or infection that it was associated with, Root-Bernstein also came tantalizingly close to inadvertently letting the cat out of the bag about the link between AIDS and CFS when he noted, "In 1986, Charles R. Rinaldo, Jr., and his co-workers demonstrated that homosexual men who seroconvert to HIV simultaneously experienced a fourfold increase in antibody titers to EBV VCA antigen (virus capsid antigen). Furthermore, they documented a direct correlation between HIV antibody titer and EBV antibody titer. The higher the one, the higher the other." (*RA* p.280) Again, inadvertently, Root-Bernstein may have uncovered the fact that AIDS was just a serious development in gay men who essentially had all the signs of "chronic mono" or "chronic fatigue syndrome." Root-Bernstein appropriately chided his fellow scientists: "Whether other viruses associated with AIDS . . . are similarly predictive of disease progression remains to be seen, since no one, as far as I can tell, has even bothered to look. This failure to look has left us in the position of assuming that HIV is the only valid measure of disease progression in AIDS, without the scientific benefit of having checked the assumption." (*RA* p.280) Checking assumptions was something that was only done on the alien non-homodemiological world of normal science.

In his chapter, "Why AIDS is Epidemic Now," Root-Bernstein may have jumped the heterosexist shark as he entered the dangerous area of speculation about the sociological underpinnings of AIDS, asserting, "To understand AIDS, we must document and understand the sociological changes in homosexuality, drug use and medical practice that have created the conditions that allowed the syndrome to explode into prominence during the past decade." (*RA* p.282) The chapter gets everything backwards. It's not that anything he says is flat out factually wrong. It's just that he misses the heterosexist context in which everything he asserts actually takes place. Every negative statement he makes about gays could be matched with a critical or negative statement about a biased heterosexual white-privileged society and the scientists who eventually entrapped gays in the bogus HIV/AIDS and "chronic fatigue syndrome is not AIDS" paradigms. Changes in homosexuality were not the only thing that needed to be discussed in order to understand the true nature of the epidemic. Changes—not good ones—in the application of society and science's white heterosexism kept up with them.

Root-Bernstein confidently notes that the "sociological manifestations of homosexuality have changed in the recent past. . . . New expressions of homosexuality concomitant with the gay liberation movement have created an unusual and new disease profile for gay men." (*RA* p.282) Root-Bernstein was clearly not applying for the position of Grand Marshal of any Gay Pride parade. While he notes, "The medical literature is quite explicit about some of these new manifestations of gay male life" (*RA* p.282)— promiscuity-related infections—he again misses the sociological fact that for every gay action there can be a heterosexist reaction and in this case "new manifestations of gay male life" were accompanied by new manifestations of heterosexist bias in science, medicine and epidemiology. Root-Bernstein certainly had a "Got-AIDS-Yet" eye for the gay guy, that focused on various aspects of gay sex that he thought were potentially linked to "AIDS." He found his smoking gun in the studies that showed "an increase in risky behavior among gay men immediately preceding the exploding in AIDS." (*RA* p.286) He also pointed to the enablers of the new "way of sex as recreation and pleasure," (*RA* p.286) namely "bath houses, backroom bars and public cruising areas." (*RA* p.286)

AIDS was—in his own epidemiological vision—the result of the sexual and recreational drug revolution. Whether it was the increase of CMV or amebiasis in gay men, *the tipping point for AIDS was gay liberation:* "AIDS became a problem for homosexual men only when rampant promiscuity, frequent anal forms of intercourse, new and sometimes physically traumatic forms of sex, and the frequent concomitants of drug use and multiple concurrent infections paved the way. As Mirko Grmek has concluded, 'American homosexuals created the conditions which, by exceeding a critical threshold, made the epidemic possible.'" (*RA* p.292) Basically this was as good as homodemiology gets. AIDS was a gay disease, so its cause ipso facto had to be intimately related to gay behavior and gay culture. It was this kind of tragic myopic epidemiological obsession that would allow the HHV-6 catastrophe to quietly simmer all over the world in all kinds of people who had never marched in a single gay liberation parade or enjoyed the diverse hedonistic pleasures that Root-Bernstein saw as the sine qua non of AIDS. Root-Bernstein doesn't say it, but it's hard not to connect the dots and conclude that the implications of his sociologically biased epidemiology that AIDS could only be stopped with a political or sociological intervention. One can only assume that in one form or another such an intervention might mean rescinding the whole gay liberation movement—or at least its sexual side.

What would never occur to Root-Bernstein was the possibility that the uneven distribution of AIDS and the apparent total safety of the heterosexual general population was a actually a mirage of groupthink, a byproduct of the political use of a heterosexist definition of AIDS that the CDC had put into play. A far more radical political and sociological analysis actually needed to be conducted *on the epidemiologists themselves* who were blind to the emerging CFS form of AIDS and the pandemic of HHV-6 that was all around while they were doing their thinking in heterosexist boxes.

Given Root-Bernstein's homodemiological approach to AIDS and his acceptance of the CDC's ground zero epidemiology, it is not surprising that he took issue with Stephen Jay Gould who wrote an alarming piece in 1987 in *The New York Times Magazine* "proclaiming heterosexual AIDS a 'natural' and therefore inevitable phenomenon." (RA p.299) This was like waving a red flag at everyone in the Duesbergian heterosexual-AIDS-is-a-myth camp. Root-Bernstein disapprovingly quotes Gould proclaiming that "the AIDS pandemic . . . may rank with nuclear weaponry as the greatest danger of our era. . . . Eventually, given the power and lability of human sexuality, it spreads outside the initial group into the general population, and now AIDS has begun its march through our own heterosexual community." (RA p.299) Gould went on to say that those infected would be "our neighbors, our lovers, our children and ourselves. AIDS is both a natural phenomenon and potentially, the greatest natural tragedy in human history." (RA p.299) Inadvertently sounding like "The Great Prophet of the chronic fatigue syndrome and Autism Epidemic," Gould was uncannily and inadvertently prescient about what was actually going on behind the CDC's biased epidemiological concoctions and sexual balkanization. He would have been spectacularly on the money if he had been referring to the HHV-6 pandemic. But HIV—not exactly.

Root-Bernstein took issue with Gould and others who in any way tried to extrapolate a picture of the future of the AIDS epidemic from what was going on in Africa. He insisted "AIDS in Africa cannot used as a model for

AIDS in Western nationals because typical sub-Saharan Africans are not comparable to Western heterosexuals in their disease load, their nutritional status, or their immunological functions." (RA p.301) This was an example of heterosexist presumptions morphing into racist presumptions. Homodemiology was becoming what I call Afrodemiology. Just as he blamed the gay revolution for AIDS in America, he noted that "Social and political revolutions are also taking their tolls on African health." (RA p.308) He pointed to Daniel B. Hrdy's notion that population movements and what Hrdy called the "sexual mixing" "of various African groups may be related to the spread of AIDS." (RA p.308) He also blamed wars in Africa which could lead to the kind of breakdown of public health infrastructure as a possible foundation for AIDS. He insisted that as far as heterosexual AIDS was concerned, "Europe and America were not Africa," (RA p.310) and "Far from presenting us with a look at the future of AIDS in North America and Europe, African heterosexuals simply confirm the fact that AIDS is a problem only for individuals who have multiple causes of immune suppression prior to, concomitant with, or independent of HIV exposure. AIDS will never become a major health threat to Americans and Western Europeans that it has become for Africans. AIDS will be a continuing problem only for individuals whose life-style, medical histories, or socioeconomic conditions predispose them to immune suppression in general." (RA p.311) This Root-Bernstein conclusion was on target only because he was blissfully unaware that whenever his fellow white American heterosexuals saw their immune systems go either south or haywire, it would be deceptively called chronic fatigue syndrome. And those unfortunate white American heterosexuals would be called crazy if they happened to notice in any way that their illness, which would be trivialized as "Yuppie Flu," was even real, significant or transmissible.

As already pointed out, like most of the Duesberg camp, Root-Bernstein was incredulous about the notion that healthy heterosexuals could ever in a million years get AIDS: "In fact, the chances that a healthy, drug free heterosexual will contract AIDS from another heterosexual are so small they were hardly worth worrying about." (RA p.313) One gets the feeling that he actually thinks it was almost literally impossible. He even doubted that cases of heterosexual cases of AIDS (as identified by the CDC) were really what they were cracked up to be. He went so far as to question the credibility of the world's most famous case of heterosexual AIDS, basketball player Magic Johnson: " . . . no one knows what risk factors Johnson did or did not have for contracting HIV other than extraordinary promiscuity. We have only his world that he contracted HIV from a woman. He has never directly stated that he never engaged in homosexual activity or used intravenous drugs." (RA p.313) In other words, he had never gotten the homodemiological third degree or the Got-AIDS-Yet? enhanced interrogation. Root-Bernstein was skeptical and asserted that "a variety of other cases touted by the government and media as heterosexually acquired AIDS cases are similarly suspect." (RA p.314)

Root-Bernstein applies the homodemiological way of sorting things out by also bringing up the possibility that the unmentionable practice of heterosexual anal sex may be a stealth factor for heterosexual AIDS in America. He argues that the female inhibition towards discussing anal sex was concealing the real reason for any supposed heterosexual AIDS. He also points out that many woman "are reticent to discuss the sharing of sexual toys such as dildos and butt plugs that may also represent modes of transmitting sexual diseases." (RA p.322) In an uncanny way, it is not too much of a stretch to suggest he was coming very close to saying that heterosexuals contracted AIDS because, although they were straight, *they had done something gay*.

One doesn't want to go too negative on Root-Bernstein, however, even if his thinking did somewhat reflect the hegemonic heterosexist culture he was part of, because at a critical time during Holocaust II, along with several others, he did play a significant part in keeping minds open enough to prevent the HIV/AIDS research elite from going completely unchallenged. He put his own reputation on the line in doing so. He also kept the door open for additional critical scientific thinking that could pick up where he left off. For those bravely standing up to a very hostile and powerful HIV/AIDS empire, his call for better science and creative scientific thinking was manna from heaven: "We must elaborate possibilities. In science, as in theater or fiction, the tension of the plot is produced by the alternative resolutions we can imagine. A plot that unfolds without suspense is boring. Similarly, in science research that can only reach one conclusion is hardly worth performing; it has no potential to yield discoveries. We want a plot that proffers alternatives. HIV has been set up as the villain of this piece, but it is still possible that we have been led [on] a merry chase away from the real culprits?" (RA p.327) He didn't realize the degree to which he was trapped in an opposite world of abnormal, totalitarian science that was driven by an agenda and a mindset that had no real interest in surprises and plot twists, discoveries and anomalies. Channeling Thomas Kuhn, he wrote, "I have previously defined scientific discovering as a process of elaborating all imaginable explanations for a phenomenon, constrained by an ever-increasing body of observation and experiment. The resulting recursive interplay of imagination and reality assures us that we have reached the correct answer." (*RA* p.328) That kind of Arendtian freedom-to-imagine was not permissible in a totalitarian world in which scientists were expected to follow HIV dogma.

When historians try to assign culpability to all the scientists who stood passively and silently on the sidelines while the medical and scientific atrocities of Holocaust II occurred, they will want to investigate the trails suggested by this statement by Root-Bernstein: "Thus, despite repeated statements by government officials that the cause of AIDS is known and that it is HIV, I can no longer find any major investigators in the field of AIDS who will defend the proposition that HIV is the only immunosuppressive agent involved in AIDS." (*RA* p.330) Whoever these scientists were, they will have to face the judgment of history when it asks why they sat on their hands and allowed the HIV mafia of Holocaust II to build a monolithic and hellish public health empire for AIDS patients and the gay community around the notion that "HIV is the only suppressive agent involved in AIDS."

It is only fair to pay special tribute to the fact that Root-Bernstein gave some rather astute, prescient attention to HHV-6 in his penultimate chapter. In discussing co-factors, he notes that even Robert Gallo had one, namely HHV-6. He quotes Gallo himself saying, "Another candidate [for an AIDS cofactor] is human herpes virus 6 (HHV-6, originally designated human B-lymphotropic virus), which has not only been identified in most patients AIDS by virus isolation, DNA amplification techniques and serological analysis, but is also predominantly tropic and cytopathic *in vitro* for CD4+ T lymphocytes . . . These observations indicate that HHV-6 might contribute directly or indirectly to the depletion of CD4+ cells in AIDS." (*RA* p.330) Root-Bernstein was far too optimistic about the flexibility and good faith of the AIDS establishment in general and Gallo in particular when he concludes, "Statements such as this one [about HHV-6] suggest that even mainstream HIV researchers are beginning to consider the possibility that HIV may not be sufficient to cause AIDS. They do not doubt that it is necessary." (*RA* p.330) To Gallo, HIV never really stopped being the "truck" that killed patients. The Nobel Prize which he felt he deserved (and still hasn't gotten) was totally dependent on that theory.

History might have been different if at this point in his rethinking Root-Bernstein had looked more critically at the psychology, sociology and politics of the world of AIDS science and epidemiology. Absent an ability to detect the presence of heterosexism and the negative effects of its cognitive bias, he was left clueless—a little like Kafka's K trying to understand what was going on in the Castle. He was sensitive to the bullheadedness of those in power but couldn't peer into the twisted souls of those in charge. He quotes the imperious Anthony Fauci, the Director of NIAID, as saying that "critiquing a dubious theory would take time away from more productive efforts." (RA p.331) And he quotes James Curran as stating unequivocally at the Amsterdam AIDS Conference in 1992 (at which it was announced that there were cases of HIV-negative AIDS), "There is not AIDS without HIV." (RA p.331) What Curran was really stubbornly saying was, "We're the Centers for Disease Control. We have the power to define disease and epidemics, and if there is HIV then we say *there has to be AIDS*, and if there is no HIV *we won't call it AIDS*. Period. End of discussion. And if you call that circular reasoning, you can just suck it up." Fauci and Curran weren't exactly stupid. They must have known where the cofactor argument might lead—to the conclusion that they had both made major contributions to the biggest scientific mistake in history. That they themselves were the final arbiters of the legitimacy of their own work is just one more factor that made AIDS a period of accountability-free abnormal and totalitarian science.

Again, Root-Bernstein seemed like he was making his own pact with the devil in giving HIV too much credibility by shaping his critique around finding cofactors for HIV rather than going all the way and asking a far more radical question of whether HIV was a total disaster-inducing red herring, the biggest scientific mistake in history. In a way, he was inadvertently helping to keep the HIV agenda alive through faint (sometimes slightly fawning) criticism. He goes out of his way to give HIV sufficient deference: "There is no doubt that HIV is highly correlated with AIDS. Correlation is not, however, proof of causation." (RA p.329) He chose to enter his own dog in the race in the form of an "HIV-plus-cofactors theory." (RA p.337) But even his theory that AIDS might be "a multifactorial, synergistic disease" kept a place for HIV as an important but not necessary opportunistic part of the disease process. He didn't fully seem to grasp that it would be *game over* for the HIV establishment if it became known that they had built their scapegoating, dystopian antigay empire around a virus that was not even necessary for AIDS. People were not jumping out of skyscrapers because they tested positive for an AIDS cofactor. People were not be arrested for transmitting an AIDS cofactor to others. People were not being turned into toxic dumps filled with AZT (and its toxic siblings) because they were infected with an AIDS cofactor.

Root-Bernstein tries to have his cake and eat it too by sticking it to Duesberg: "I believe that Duesberg is wrong in ignoring the role of HIV in AIDS. It is certainly highly correlated with the syndrome (even given the methodological sleight of hand involved in defining the syndrome by the presence of the putative causative agent prior to definitive demonstration of causation) . . . . It is just as big a mistake to ignore the potential role of HIV in AIDS as it is to ignore the roles of all other immunosuppressive agents that affect AIDS patients." (*RA* p.343) The AIDS establishment was not shaking in its boots about the latter charge. The AIDS empire was not being built on the premise that HIV *contributed* to AIDS like a wide array of other immunosuppressive agents. HIV was being packaged as the Gay Andromeda Strain. It was an evil and inexorable agent. Those infected with it carried an evil germ and were capable of doing a great deal of damage to society with the venereally-transmitted agent, meaning that those people's very sexual identities were being permanently tied to the single evil virus.

In many ways, the notions that Peter Duesberg proffered about AIDS were not any less heterosexist than Root-Bernstein's, but with far more political sensitivity than Root-Bernstein, Duesberg grasped the personal implications for anyone who got caught in the labyrinth of epidemiological fraud and ended up labeled HIV positive, the virtual medical Yellow Star (or more accurately, a Pink Triangle) with all the perks that went with it. They weren't just being labeled "cofactor positive." Peter Duesberg had the kind of empathetic x-ray vision that could see the human toll the scientific mistake (or fraud) of HIV was taking.

For all we know, Root-Bernstein may have thought that his was a kind of big tent compromise position that could bring the anti-HIV camp back to the scientific table with the growing HIV establishment so as to develop a new synthesis of both positions, but it was all for naught regardless of his good intentions. The AIDS establishment had bet their professional and financial lives on HIV and Duesberg thought HIV was a non-negotiable crock and that was that. And while all of these scientists fiddled with arguments about HIV, Rome was burning with HHV-6 and its family of viruses.

Root-Bernstein ends his important book by asking how so many scientists could be so wrong about something and reminds his readers that "Science, despite its elusive goal of objective truth, is just as human and just as fallible as any other human activity." (*RA* p.350) It is his belief that oversimplification and gullibility have contributed to the mistake of thinking HIV is the cause of AIDS. He asserts, "authority—even wishful thinking—is just as powerful and prevalent in science and medicine as it is in any other sphere of human endeavor." (RA p.353) He also points out the scandalous and unbelievable fact that studies have shown that "physicians are perhaps the most authority oriented of all professionals. They are evaluated in medical school not on the basis of their critical thinking skills, their creativity, or their independence but their ability to learn quickly, to memorize well, to act prudently, and to be able to quote authority extensively." (RA p.353) They would clearly also make good priests—which is what some of them seemed like during Holocaust II. He goes to the tragic heart of the matter when he writes, "There can be no breakthroughs without research, but breakthrough research is not possible when conformity is rewarded and skeptical inquiry punished. AIDS may continue to plague modern society, just as other preventable infections such a puerperal fever plagued our forebears, because of the closemindedness of the very physicians whose job it is to diagnose, treat, and prevent these diseases." (RA p.354) He didn't know the half of it. In the solace of his certainty that these mistakes didn't put the heterosexual general population at risk, he thought he was throwing life rafts at pathetic, drowning risk groups from a boat that couldn't sink. He didn't know he was standing on the white heterosexual Titanic.

As with Duesberg and Kary Mullis, one must express gratitude that he joined those who spoke out against AZT and similar treatments: "One caveat concerning long-term prophylaxis for AIDS is in order. As I have pointed out repeatedly, chronic use of antibiotics can lead to immune suppression. . . . There are, however, almost no long-term studies of the effects of chronic exposure to the vast majority of drugs that might be used prophylactically in AIDS. . . . We do not want to be in the position of saying that we cured the patient but the treatment killed him." (RA p.337) We don't? We didn't? Could have fooled us. He caught the real tragedy of blaming the wrong agent for AIDS when he pointed out that "It may prove easier to stop a mycoplasmal or cytomegalovirus infection [or any infection that be part of the mutifactorial mix in AIDS] than to stop HIV." (RA p.357)

It is once again disquieting to note how close to the truth of the HHV-6 catastrophe Root-Bernstein actually got and how much help he could have been if he had stayed with the issue—as focused and critical as he was in his book—for another decade. Thinking way outside the AIDS box, he even theorized that scientists could have gotten the whole orthodox paradigm of immunosuppression in AIDS *backwards* when he speculated that "One very odd possibility is also raised by alternative theories of AIDS, particularly by the theories that incorporate autoimmunity as a major event in the prognosis of the disease. Immunosuppressive drugs may actually benefit AIDS patients." (*RA* p.358) Such a radical change in the AIDS paradigm would have caused what Kuhn refers to as a "visual gestalt shift," but that was simply not allowed in the totalitarian, abnormal, paralyzed world of AIDS science. Without fully realizing it, Root-Bernstein was tilting at political windmills when he wrote, "In the meantime, various aspects of medical practice must change to accommodate the possibility that HIV is not the sole agent responsible for AIDS." (*RA* p.358) To which one could hear every member of the HIV establishment thinking, "Over our dead bodies." There would absolutely be no dialing back on the AIDS paradigm or agenda. Rethinking was for "denialists." HIV would never ever be considered "no more than a serious warning that a patient has multiple risks that need to be ferreted out and controlled and corrected." (*RA* p.358.) He might just as well have proposed that homeopathy be applied to AIDS. There was no way that the crown jewel of homodemiology (and Afrodemiology) was going to be abandoned. Its totalitarian power to stigmatize, control and for some to make a lot of money and advance careers was not something to be given up without a vicious fight to the death.

Like a good Kuhnian, Root-Bernstein thought that the answers to AIDS might come from unexpected sources, from people not at the center of the reigning establishment that controlled the shape of the official paradigm: "I would not be surprised if the most important innovators in AIDS research and treatment turn out to be peripheral members of the research and treatment communities." (*RA* p.363) Following the rules of abnormal science, AIDS research was the enemy of true innovation. AIDS was dogmatic and innovation was heresy and worthy of inquisition. To cross the AIDS leadership was to become a peripheral member of the research and treatment communities.

Near the end of his book the very earnest Root-Bernstein makes a statement full of laugh-out-loud irony for any student of Holocaust II: "We need to solve the social, economic, health education, and medical care problems that create the conditions that permit AIDS to develop in the first place." (*RA* p.368) Fair enough, but the number one problem hidden in that politically correct smorgasbord is something that Root-Bernstein was himself an (albeit relatively decent) ambassador of: white heterosexism. White heterosexism may have had social and economic cofactors in the creation of Holocaust II, but it still was the sine qua non. White heterosexism is what held the AIDS quilt—so to speak—together. And ultimately it would also blindly hold the CFS and autism quilts together.

Root-Bernstein closes his book by asserting that "The only path to the truth is to continue questioning—even things that are taken to be undeniable facts." (*RA* p.373) Given that we are now in the middle of an HHV-6 spectrum catastrophe which is potentially affecting everyone immunologically, neurologically and in a variety of other ways and manifesting itself as an alphabet soup of AIDS, CFS, MS, autism, cancer, Morgellons and God knows what else, he may want to question some of the ground zero data and epidemiology that led to his belief that *the general population had nothing to worry about* where the virtually impossible lightning strike of AIDS was concerned. One day he just might want to write a sequel to *Rethinking AIDS* called "Rethinking My Rethinking of AIDS."

Serge Lang

The Righteous Mathematician

Serge Lang (1927-2005) was one of the most distinguished elder academic statesman in the group intellectuals and scientists that challenged the science of HIV. A mathematician known for his accomplishments in number theory and as the author of numerous graduate level mathematics text books, he taught at the University of Chicago and Columbia University. He was Professor Emeritus at Yale University at the time of his death. He was very active in the Vietnam anti-war movement and spent a great deal of time challenging the misuse of science and mathematics and identifying the spread of misinformation on a number of issues. Lang was rewarded for his interest in the Duesbergian criticism of HIV and for speaking out on the questionable scientific procedures of the HIV establishment, by having his distinguished career in mathematics framed by the same dirty little Orwellian trick used on other HIV critics: he was labeled an "AIDS denialist," by that paragon of sober objectivity, Wikipedia.

As Lang surveyed the manner in which AIDS research was being conducted and the outrageous way that Duesberg was being treated, he was appalled and feared for the integrity of science itself. In 1984, his long critique of the HIV/AIDS theory was published in the Fall issue of *Yale Scientific*. He opened his piece by pointing out the sleight of hand involved in the naming of the virus *only associated* with AIDS which was called "Human Immunodeficiency Virus" before adequate evidence had been gathered to show that it actually deserved that title. Which, of course it didn't. Lang's critical vision of what was transpiring in AIDS was quite damming: " . . . to an extent that undermines classical standards of science, some purported scientific results concerning 'HIV' and 'AIDS' have been handled by press releases, by misinformation, manipulating the media and people at large." Much of Lang's analysis of AIDS science supports the contention that AIDS could best be described as science at its most abnormal. But he stayed away from the matter of the motivation behind the breakdown of science, asserting, "I am not here concerned with intent but with scientific standards, especially the ability to tell the difference between a fact, an opinion, a hypothesis, and a hole in the ground." Even though Lang steered clear of digging into the bigotry that motivated and unified the whole pseudoscientific enterprise, he did make it abundantly clear that there was something *not kosher* about the field of HIV/AIDS research. He argued that there wasn't even a proper definition of "AIDS" and "thus a morass about HIV and AIDS has been created." Lang called the established view of AIDS "dogma" and he was horrified by the way people who dared to challenge the "dogma" were being treated, noting that critics were unfairly being maligned by being called "flatearthers" or told that by just asking questions or being skeptical they were themselves threats to the public health. He was very sensitive to the emotional blackmail that was a staple in the AIDS establishment's psychological armamentarium.

In the *Yale Scientific* piece, Lang argued that "the public at large are not properly informed" and in order for them to know what was really happening, people had to turn to sources outside of the official scientific media. He thought that the way AIDS misinformation was being spread was itself an important issue that needed a focused study. He charged that the official scientific press had failed miserably by obstructing legitimate dissent and that not only would the public lose "trust in the scientific establishment," but people would not be "warned of practices which may be dangerous to their health." As we now know, he was only seeing the tip of the pseudoscientific iceberg.

Lang reiterated the Mullis contention that there were no papers that provided proof that HIV is the cause of AIDS, and no serious HIV animal model for the disease. He was very concerned about the unreliable tests for HIV: "The blood test for HIV does not determine directly the presence of the virus." The test cross-reacted with numerous other diseases. He argued that the AIDS numbers coming out of Africa were based on faulty testing. In terms of the HHV-6 catastrophe that everyone was willfully blind to at the time, it is interesting to note Lang's argument that "there exist thousands of Americans who have AIDS-defining diseases but are HIV negative." Had he said millions, we might be calling him a prophet of the HHV-6 spectrum catastrophe. The argument for HIV was made even worse by the fact that there were "hundreds of thousands who test HIV positive but have not developed AIDS-defining diseases." He accused the CDC of playing games with numbers to support their official image of the epidemic. He was also critical of the CDC's circular definition of AIDS that made it look like there was a 100% correlation between HIV and AIDS in the public's mind. He argued that HIV positivity might "be merely a marker rather than a cause for whatever disease is involved." He was intrigued by the Duesbergian recreational drug hypothesis, but remained open-minded. He wrote, "I have no definitive answer. I merely question the line upheld up to now by the biomedical establishment, and repeated uncritically in the press, that 'HIV is the virus that causes AIDS.'" He felt that because most scientists treated HIV=AIDS as a given, "some scientists try to fit experimental data into this postulate, actually without success." They succeed even when they fail: when the so-called AIDS virus doesn't meet expectations, Lang notes that it is then called "enigmatic" without anyone going back to basics and questioning the science and logic that form the foundation upon which it stands.

Lang was troubled by the unwillingness of the establishment to fund research into alternative hypotheses about AIDS causation—particularly Duesberg's recreational drug hypothesis. He felt that the evidence that the recreational inhalant, "poppers" (amyl nitrite), played a role in AIDS via the development of Kaposi's sarcoma, was compelling enough that it didn't deserve the cold financial shoulder it was consistently getting from those in charge of the governmental funding of AIDS research

In the Yale Scientific piece, Lang also criticized "establishment scientists who have tried, so far mostly successfully, to keep reports questioning the establishment dogma about HIV out of the mainstream press." The Pacific Division of the American Association for the Advancement of Science organized a symposium for June 21, 1994 called "The Role of HIV in AIDS: Why There is Still a Controversy." Lang reported that the AAAS "has come under fire from U.S. AIDS researchers and public health officials" and the symposium was almost cancelled. An article about the symposium in the journal, Nature, quoted a professor from Harvard as saying that the people involved were "fringe" people. David Baltimore was quoted as saying, "This is a group of people who have denied the scientific facts. There is no question at all that HIV is the cause of AIDS. Anyone who gets up publicly and says the opposite is encouraging people to risk their lives." Again, the emotional blackmail of what today would be called the "concern trolls of HIV/AIDS."

Lang reported that while the symposium was finally held, Nature made a point of not covering it. Lang sharply noted, "Nature's readers are not given evidence on which to base an informed or independent judgment. Thus does Nature manipulate its readers." And thus did that esteemed journal help enable the abnormal science of Holocaust II.

Lang captures the manner in which the media was manipulated during the AIDS era in his description of a study meant to demolish Duesberg's drug hypothesis: "A piece, 'Does drug use cause AIDS?' by M.S. Ascher, H.W. Shepherd., W. Winkelstein Jr. and E. Vittinghoff was published in the Nature issue of 11 March 1993. This piece was published as a 'Commentary.' About a week before publication, nature issued a press release concerning this piece headlined: 'DRUG USE DOES NOT CAUSE AIDS.' The press release concluded: 'These findings seriously undermine the argument put forward by Dr. Peter Duesberg, of the University of California at Berkley, that drug consumption causes AIDS.'" Lang noted that Duesberg was blind-sided because the press was notified and was asking him for a response even before he had even had a chance to see the forthcoming piece. Lang wrote bitterly, "Thus Nature and the authors of the article use the media to manipulate public opinion before their article had been submitted to scientific scrutiny by other scientists (other than possible referees), and especially by Duesberg who is principally concerned."

Lang attacked the press release, writing that it made several misrepresentations including the manner in which the sample of men studied was gathered: " . . . the press release suppressed the additional information that the sampling came from a definite segment of San Francisco households." Lang's analysis of what the Ascher group called "a rigorously controlled epidemiological model for the evaluation of aetiological hypotheses" pointed to numerous flaws that made the study look like a bad joke—which was par for the course in the world of AIDS science. He notes that predictably, The New York Times which, with the help of Lawrence Altman, a reporter who was a former CDC employee, was the world's most prestigious echo chamber for the government's AIDS research, ran with the ball. An article by Gina Kolata called "Debunking doubts that H.I.V. causes AIDS," propagated "the misinformation of the [Nature] press release and of the 'Commentary.'"

Lang's sense of scientific standards was offended by the whole picture of AIDS science that he saw: "I take no position here on the relative merits of the AIDS virus hypothesis or the AIDS drug hypothesis (in whatever form they may be formulated). I do take a position against the announcement of purported scientific results via superficial and defective press releases, and before scientists at large have had a chance to evaluate the scientific merits of such results are purportedly based." What Lang didn't fully understand was that this kind of propagandistic manipulation of truth was actually business as usual in the totalitarian abnormal science of Holocaust II.

One of the more amusingly outrageous aspects of Ascher's 'Commentary' in Nature, appears at the end of the piece: "The energies of Duesberg and his followers could be better applied to unraveling the enigmatic mechanism of the HIV pathogenesis of AIDS." To this patronizing bums rush Lang responded, "I find it presumptuous and objectionable for scientists to tell others where energies 'could better be applied.' Scientific standards as I have known them since I was a freshman at Caltech require that some energies be applied to scrutinize data on which experiments are based, in documenting the accuracy of the data, its significance, its completeness, and to determine whether conclusions allegedly based on these data are legitimate or not." Lang didn't realize that Ascher was part of a political bandwagon driven by social forces which Lang, as brilliant as he was, was not interested in or perhaps even capable of fully fathoming.

In his piece in Yale Scientific, Lang also raised the issue of the role of other viruses in AIDS, stating, "No hypothesis can be dismissed a priori. It is still a possibility that some viruses other than HIV sometimes cause some of the diseases listed under the "AIDS" umbrella by the CDC." One of those he mentions in the piece is HHV-6. He clearly was intrigued by the paradox of a supposedly ubiquitous and usually (or also supposedly) harmless virus also being associated with pneumonitis in compromised hosts. He inadvertently went right to the heart of the political and scientific problems that HHV-6 would be entangled with in the years ahead when he wrote, "Here we meet typical examples of rising questions: whether there is merely an 'association' between a virus and some disease, or whether a virus is a cause, and if so how. It is then a problem to make experiments to determine whether a given virus is merely a passenger virus, whether it lies dormant, and if it is awakened (how?). Whether it merely shows its presence by testing positive in various ways (antibodies?), or whether it is or becomes harmful (how?), under certain circumstances (which?)." He had unknowingly stumbled into the tragic intellectual fog of the HHV-6 catastrophe, the biomedical tragedy that the Orwellian propaganda about HIV was obscuring.

One of the more curious episodes in the struggles of the Duesbergian camp concerns Serge Lang's encounter with Richard Horton, the then youngish editor of The Lancet who was pretty much in the bag for the HIV establishment. It is described in Challenges, Lang's book of essays. It is a must-read for anyone interested in the slovenliness of the intellectual community during Holocaust II. Horton had written a 9,000 word review article, "Truth and Heresy about AIDS" which was critical of Duesberg and published in the New York Review of Books (May 23, 1996). In response, Lang submitted a letter as long as Horton's book review itself to NYBR but it was rejected. Lang's unpublished letter charged that Horton's review gave "a false impression of scientific scholarship" and did not convey to the readers the complexity of the debate about HIV and AIDS. Horton had reviewed two books by Duesberg and one book which was a collection of 27 articles called AIDS: Virus—or Drug Induced?, which included two articles by Lang. Horton completely ignored the more important of Lang's two articles—the one we just discussed that was reprinted from Yale Scientific. Not only did Horton ignore Lang's detailed critique of HIV, but he also ignored everyone published in the collection except Duesberg, contributing to the image of Duesberg that the HIV establishment had cleverly manufactured and marketed, namely the fringy lone gunman: Lang wrote, "Horton mentioned Duesberg repeatedly as a critic of the established view, but by not referring to the multiple articles in the . . . collection he made it appear as if Duesberg is more isolated than he actually is in raising objections." In addition to criticizing Horton for personalizing the issue rather than engaging in scientific discussion, Lang criticized Horton for not informing his readers about misinformation the government had put out about AIDS and for ignoring legitimate questions about the reliability or credibility of the HIV test. He suggested that Horton had fudged "the issue about relationships between AIDS (whatever it is), HIV and other viruses such as a persistent herpes virus." (The truth about the looming HHV-6 catastrophe was so close to Lang that it could have bitten him.)

Lang pointed out that Duesberg was getting the silent treatment from Horton's own publication, The Lancet, where he "has not been allowed to publish longer pieces, [other than letters] either as a scientific article, or as a 'Viewpoint.'" Lang also attacked Horton for resorting to what could be called "emotional public health blackmail" when he pointed to the fact that Horton wrote in his review, "Duesberg's arguments take him into dangerous territory. For if HIV is not the cause of AIDS, then every public health injunction about the need for safe sex becomes meaningless." Dangerous territory? (Certainly dangerous territory for those behind the Potemkin HIV paradigm that hid the truth about Holocaust II.) Lang held that Horton's warning "bypasses the specific objections and questions, and draws an invalid extreme conclusion." As was typical throughout Holocaust II, every time anyone asked a critical question about HIV it was as though they had taken a bullhorn and were shouting out encouragements to the public to run wild and naked in the street without condoms. It often came across as a veiled, patronizing, heterosexist assault against the dignity and intelligence of the gay community. Remarks like those made AIDS look like a public health campaign that was more concerned about behavioral control than truth—which in many ways it was.

New York Review of Books published an exchange of letters between Duesberg and Horton on August 8, 1996. Among a number of things Lang was critical of in Horton's letter, he was especially incensed by Horton's challenge that "If Duesberg seriously believes there is nothing to fear from HIV, he can easily prove it. If Duesberg seriously believes that HIV is harmless, let him inject himself with a suspension of the virus." Lang asserted, "Horton's logic is deficient on several counts. First, self-experimentation by Duesberg would not 'prove' (let alone 'easily prove') anything about a virus which is supposed to take ten years to achieve is pathogenic effects. Second, the negation of one extreme is not the extreme of opposite type. Here may be something to fear from poppers (amyl nitrites) or AZT, as well as HIV." Serge Lang perceptively honed in on the very peculiar debating style that characterized Holocaust II when he wrote, "Horton's reply with the above challenge to Duesberg pushed the discussion to extremes in an unscientific and ad hominem manner. He turns the discussion to considerations of beliefs, rather than facts ('If Duesberg seriously believes . . .'). But it is not a question what 'Duesberg believes.' What's involved scientifically are, among other things: the possibility of making certain experiments (some of them on animals); whether certain data (epidemiological or laboratory) are valid (e.g. properly gathered and reported); whether interpretations of the data are valid; the extent to which certain hypotheses are compatible with the data; and whether scientific objections to specific scientific articles are legitimately or substantially answered, if answered at all."

There was a second exchange between Horton and Duesberg in NYRB. According to Lang, "Horton devoted the greater part of his second reply to the ad hominem challenge, and some history of self-experimentation. Thus Horton compounded the problems raised by his ad hominem attack. Self-experimentation is something which a scientist may offer unprompted, as has sometimes been done in the past. Whether to do so or not is for each scientist to decide individually. I object to other scientists putting pressure for self-experimentation especially in a journalistic context." On 2 August 1996, Lang submitted a letter to the editors of the New York Review which was about 500 words long. The letter was rejected. Lang was so disturbed by Horton's unprofessional suggestion of self-experimentation that he submitted his rejected letter as a half-page advertisement to New York Review with a check for $3,500 to cover the cost. The editor returned the check and agreed to publish the letter.

Lang was incensed that NYRB had not published several other letters from scientists defending Duesberg. The New York Review's behavior shocked Lang who had been both a contributor and an admirer of the publication's integrity and intellectual legacy. He summarized its importance: "With its world-wide circulation of 120,000, it is very influential in the academic and intellectual community. Members of these communities rely on the New York Review for information they cannot get easily elsewhere. Flaws in the New York Review editorial judgment are therefore very serious." (Lang would live to see the New York Review betray its ideal even more egregiously years later when they attacked South Africa's brave HIV critic, Thabo Mbeki.)

Lang wrote about the pseudoscience of HIV/AIDS like someone whose scientific heart was breaking. In the Horton/NYRB piece he wistfully quotes Richard Feynman who called for scientists to have "a kind of scientific integrity, a principle of scientific thought that corresponds to a kind of utter honesty—a kind of leaning over backwards. For example, if you're doing an experiment, you should report everything that you think might make it invalid—not only what you think is right about it: other causes that could possibly explain your results; and things you thought of that you've eliminated by some other experiment, and how they worked—to make sure the other fellow can tell they have been eliminated. Details that could throw doubt on your interpretation must be given, if you know anything at all wrong, or possibly wrong—to explain it. If you make a theory, for example, and advertise it, or put it out, then you must also put down all the facts that disagree with it, as well as those that agree with it. In summary, the idea is to try to give all the information to help others to judge the value of your contribution; not just the information that leads to judgment in one particular direction or another."

Feynman's good faith vision of science operating at its best was like the opposite world of AIDS and Holocaust II. Richard Horton was one of the powerful little princes of that opposite world and the very principled Serge

Lang's unflappable, stubborn and inspiring confrontation with Horton on the intellectual world stage during the depressing days of Holocaust II reminds one of what Hannah Arendt wrote about Karl Jaspers in Men in Dark Times: "It was self-evident that he would remain firm in the midst of catastrophe. . . . There is something fascinating about a man's being inviolable, untemptable, unswayable." (Men in Dark Times p.76) But even the inviolable, untemptable, and unswayable Serge Lang could not stop the catastrophe of Holocaust II.

Rebecca Culshaw

The Whistleblower Who Almost Nailed It

Hopefully, when filmmakers finally start to realize how many rich narrative possibilities there are in the real history of Holocaust II, Rebecca's Culshaw's dramatic awakening to the dark nature of HIV/AIDS science or pseudoscience will be recognized as a compelling story that deserves to be a movie by itself. Culshaw received her Ph.D. in 2002 for work constructing mathematical models of HIV infection, a field of study she had entered in 1996. In an essay, "Why I Quite HIV," (available online) she said that her entire adolescence and adult life "has been overshadowed by the belief in a deadly, sexually transmittable pathogen and the attendant fear of intimacy and lack of trust that belief engenders." During her work on AIDS she came to realize "that there is good evidence that the entire basis for this theory is wrong. AIDS, it seems is not a disease so much as a sociopolitical construct that few people understand and even fewer question."

At one point earlier in her life, she was led to believe that she had contracted "AIDS" and she took an HIV test. She spent two weeks waiting for the results, convinced she was going to die and blaming herself for whatever she might have done to cause the development. She tested negative and "vowed not to take more risks."

Ten years later when she was a graduate student analyzing models of HIV and the immune system, she was surprised to discover that virtually every mathematical model of HIV infection she studied was unrealistic. She concluded that the "biological assumptions on which the models were based varied from author to author." She was also puzzled by the stories of long-term survivors of AIDS and the fact that all of them seemed to have one thing in common—very healthy lifestyles. It made her suspect that "being HIV-positive didn't necessarily mean you would ever get AIDS."

When she ran across the writing of one of Peter Duesberg's supporters, David Rasnick, it all began to make more sense to her. Rasnick had written an article on AIDS and the corruption of modern science which resonated with her own troubling academic experience. She found an intellectual soulmate when she read Rasnick's assertion that the more he "examined HIV, the less it made sense that this largely inactive, barely detectable virus could cause such devastation." Culshaw continued to work on HIV, however, and published four papers on HIV from a mathematical modeling perspective. She wrote, "I justified my contributions to a theory I wasn't convinced of by telling myself these were purely theoretical, mathematical constructs, never to be applied to the real world. I supposed, in some sense also, I wanted to keep an open mind." But eventually she reached a breaking point on HIV.

She had been taught early in her career that clear definitions were important and as far as she could tell, the definition of AIDS was anything but. AIDS was not "even a consistent entity." She was concerned that the definition of AIDS in the early 1980s was a surveillance tool that bore no resemblance to the AIDS of the current time. She was troubled by the fact that the CDC constantly changed the definition, that people could be diagnosed when there was no evidence of clinical disease and the fact that the leading cause of death of HIV positives was from liver failure caused by the AIDS treatments (protease inhibitors) themselves.

The epidemiology completely puzzled her. The fact that the number of HIV positives in the U.S. "has remained constant at one million" seemed to make no sense. She wrote, "It is deeply confusing that a virus thought to have been brought to the AIDS epicenters of New York, San Francisco and Los Angeles in the early 1970s could possibly have spread so rapidly at first, yet have stopped spreading as soon as testing began." She had entered the gates of the opposite world of totalitarian, Orwellian, abnormal science where the numbers of positives could remain constant because their origins were political and not based on factuality.

She also thought that the theories about how HIV destroyed t-cells didn't add up and was disturbed that after so many years of study there was still no "biological consensus" about the manner in which HIV did its dirty work. Culshaw was frustrated by the fact that "there are no data to support the hypothesis that HIV kills cells. It doesn't in the test tube. It mostly just sits there, as it does in people—if it can be found at all." The shocking fact that Gallo had originally only found the virus in 26 of 72 AIDS patients was also a dramatic strike against the notion that it was the cause of AIDS.

Culshaw found further support for her growing skepticism in the testing for HIV which relies on antibody tests rather than searching for the virus itself because "there exists no test for the actual virus." The fact that so-called viral load tests relied on sophisticated PCR techniques that had never actually been tested against a gold standard of HIV itself made the whole enterprise of HIV testing look like a cruel and dangerous farce. The fact that the criteria for a positive result for the antibody varied from country to country also undermined the credibility of the HIV tests. Culshaw concluded, "I have come to sincerely believe that the HIV tests do immeasurably more harm than good, due to their astounding lack of specificity and standardization. . . . A negative test may not be accurate (whatever that means), but a positive one can create utter havoc and destruction in a person's life—all for a virus that most likely does absolutely nothing. I do not feel it is going too far to say that these tests ought to be banned for diagnostic purposes."

She indicted thousands of her intellectual and professional colleagues when she wrote, "After ten years involved in the academic side of HIV research, as well as in the academic world at large, I truly believe that the blame for the universal, unconditional, faith-based acceptance of such a flawed theory fall on those among us who have actively endorsed a completely unproven hypothesis in the interests of furthering our careers."

Culshaw summed up her thoughts on AIDS in a brief but brilliant book, Science Sold Out, which was published two years later by North Atlantic Books. The book is so tautly written and sizzles with so much moral outrage that one could say that she was the Thomas Paine (or one of them) of Holocaust II. She opens the book with an anecdotal challenge to HIV from her personal life: "The boyfriend of a woman I work with died suddenly this year from a raging infection. He became very ill, and his immune system collapsed, unable to handle the infection, and he died. He was not HIV-positive, but if he had been he would have been an AIDS case." (SSO p.viii) While most of the Duesbergians focused mainly on what was diagnosed mistakenly as AIDS—diagnoses they disagreed with—it is interesting that she begins her little masterpiece with a case that might inadvertently have pointed to a far darker implication of the CDC and the AIDS establishment's misguided epidemiology: that they were missing the real epidemic and as a result an unknown number of people were dying mysteriously.

None of the arguments in her book were completely new, but her presentation was a tour de force. It was full of the most righteous indignation of any of the critical books on HIV and AIDS, with the possible exception of the work of John Lauritsen, who I have discussed at length in my book, The Chronic Fatigue Syndrome Epidemic Cover-up. She also brought an astute political and sociological analysis to the table that helped make what we've called Holocaust II more understandable as a historic event: "AIDS has become so mired in emotion, hysteria and politics that it is no longer primarily a health issue. AIDS has been transported out of the realm of public and personal health and into a strange new world in which pronouncements by powerful governmental officials are taken as gospel, and no one remembers when, a few years later, these pronouncements turn out to be false." (SSO p.4) That the scientific establishment had been so quick to accept the HIV theory was shocking. The willingness of the public to trust proclamations from the government on the issue was also unsettling. She made it her job to try and sort out the sociological reasons for the rush to judgment and the bizarre and stubborn anti-scientific refusal to entertain second and third opinions on the matter.

As Culshaw looked back at the history of AIDS, she saw a disturbing pattern that made it appear as if scientists were making everything up haphazardly and illogically as they went along: "Science, of course, is meant to be self-correcting, but it seems to be endemic in HIV research that, rather than continuously building an accumulating body of secure knowledge with only occasional missteps, the bulk of the structure gets knocked down every three to four years, replaced by yet another hypothesis, standard of care, or definition of what exactly, AIDS really is. This new structure eventually gets knocked down in the same fashion." (SSO p.11) Inadvertently, she was actually sensing the totalitarian, abnormal, deviant, ad hoc, a posteriori nature of criminal, scientific opposite world she had stumbled into. She could grasp the hypocritical and dishonest nature of the infernal game that was being played in the name of science when she wrote, "Even more disturbing is the fact that HIV researchers continuously claim that certain papers' results are out of date, yet have absolutely no hesitation in citing the entire body of scientific research on HIV as massive overwhelming evidence in favor of HIV. They can't have it both ways, yet this is what they try to do." (SSO p.12) In the opposite world of AIDS science meant having everything every-which-way all of the time.

As Culshaw wrestles with the question of why so many scientists could be so wrong for so long, she points out that, contrary to the HIV establishment's propaganda, a significant number of scientists actually did join Duesberg in his skepticism and dissent. One of the more interesting scientists she mentions is Rodney Richards, "a chemist who worked for the company Amgen developing the first HIV antibody tests [who] contends that the antibody tests are at best measuring a condition called hypergammaglobulinemia . . . a word that simply means too many antibodies to too many things." (SSO p.13) (This—unknown to Culshaw—may have been the major clue that CFS and AIDS were manifestations of the same hypergammaglobulinemia epidemic, and explain why both groups, in addition to testing positive for HHV-6 also tested positive for retroviral activity due to the hypergamma-globulinemia.)

Culshaw agreed with the HIV/AIDS critic David Rasnick, that a contributing factor in the reign of scientific error was an "epidemic of low standards that is infecting all of academic scientific research." (SSO p.13) She argued that "it was almost inevitable that a very significant scientific mistake was going to be made." (SSO p.15) Culshaw was very critical of the AIDS establishment's refusal to publicly discuss and defend its science: "If the AIDS establishment is so convinced of the validity of what they say, they should have no fear of a public, adjudicated debate between the major orthodox and dissenting scientists, and the scrutiny of such a debate by the scientific community." (SSO p.17) Scrutiny to AIDS researchers was like sunlight to vampires.

Culshaw was just as flabbergasted at the very strange moment that HTLV-III was transformed politically into the "AIDS virus" as the rest of the Duesbergians: "It was sometime in 1985 that HIV conspicuously went from 'the virus associated with AIDS' to the 'virus that causes AIDS,' squelching debate in the scientific arena. What changed? What happened to make scientists come to such certainty? If you look at the actual papers you'll see quite clearly that the answer is nothing." (SSO p.19) In other words, this life-and-death matter was settled by politics and public relations rather than anything resembling Kuhnian normal science. HIV/AIDS, according to Culshaw, then became a "machine" that kept moving despite all efforts at dissent. It had an evil life of its own.

Culshaw focuses on the protease inhibitor part of the tragedy of Holocaust II by walking her readers through the chronology of the questionable science that the so-called "cocktails" were based on. Papers by David Ho (Time's Man of the Year) and Xiping Wei that were published in Nature inspired an approach to treating AIDS of "Hit hard, hit early," that was to turn the hoodwinked and cheering gay community into one big deadly iatrogenic AIDS cocktail party. The only problem with the cocktails, according to Culshaw, was that "few people are aware that the conclusions" that supported the approach "were based on very poorly constructed mathematical models," and "to make matters worse, the statistical analysis were poorly done and the graphs were presented in such a way as to lead the reader to believe something different from what the data supported." (SSO p.20) Deceptive, abnormal science was alive and well during the David Ho HIV/AIDS cocktail era. Ho's slovenly work was called "ground breaking" by Sir John Maddox of Nature who said that it provided a compelling reason that the critics of HIV (especially Peter Duesberg) should "recant." (SSO p.20) A perfect word for the AIDS Inquisition.

Culshaw saw the circular logic game of molding data to fit the theory being played out in AIDS in the mathematics-based papers that were used to justify the protease inhibitor era, noting that "such tactics by definition, are excellent at maintaining a façade of near-perfect correlation between HIV and AIDS and of providing seeming convincing explanations of HIV pathogenesis." (SSO p.21) Once again the public relations requirements of the HIV/AIDS paradigm were being serviced by the fancy footwork of abnormal science. The inexorable nature of Holocaust II is captured in the fact that even though "the Ho/Wei papers have been debunked by both establishment and dissenting researchers on biological as well as mathematical grounds," the therapies that were concoctions based on that discredited science "are used to this day." (SSO p.21) The reader stares in helpless horror at the atrocities of the HIV/AIDS era as Culshaw reiterates that " . . . a large population of people have been, and continue to be, treated on the basis of a theory that is unsupportable." (SSO p.21) Culshaw's moral outrage is riveting: "You might imagine that people might feel an urge to discuss the manner in which the papers got published and whether other such mistakes have happened since that time. You might imagine that the failure of the peer-review process to detect such patently inept research would send off alarm bells within the HIV-research community. You would be wrong." (SSO p.21) Standard operating procedure in Holocaust II.

Without calling it virtual iatrogenic genocide, she indicts a whole generation of clinicians who continued to base their treatment of patients on Ho and Wei: "HIV researchers know the Ho/Wei papers are wrong, yet they continue along the clinical path charted by the papers. They know that the quantitative use of PCR has never been validated, yet they continue to use viral load to make clinical decisions." (SSO p.21) As we have said, it took a village of professionals to create Holocaust II.

One thinks about the proverbial story of the drunk looking for his car keys in the parking lot under a light far from his actual car because that's the only place there is light—when one reads this analysis from Culshaw about a scientist's discovery in the first so-called AIDS patients: "Upon measuring their t-cells, a subset of the immune system, he found that in all five men they were depleted. What is quite curious about this discovery is that the technology to count t-cells had only just been perfected."(SSO p.23) This is yet another way of saying that epidemics never get a second chance to make a first impression. Shiny new toys can create erroneous new paradigms in science.

Culshaw gets to the crux of the AIDS establishment's mistake by noting that they rushed to judgment on HIV and then were then trapped and had to trim data and cook the books (like the frantic maintainers of a threatened Ponzi scheme) in order to fit their stubborn theories to match disparities in the growing number of people they were designating as having AIDS: "As the definition expanded and as it became more and more clear that HIV did not do at all what it was purported to do—that is, kill CD4 t-cells by any detectable method—researchers began to invent more and more convoluted explanations for why their theory was correct." (SSO p.24) Good money was constantly thrown after bad. Of course, from this writer's perspective, had they also expanded the definition so much as to include the chronic fatigue syndrome epidemic, things might have miraculously straightened themselves out and HHV-6's role in the hypergammaglobulinemia epidemic might have become painfully obvious.

Channeling Thomas Kuhn, Culshaw is all too old fashioned and normal-science-ish when she so reasonably writes, "The logical scientific thing to have done would have been to notice their original disease designation did not accurately identify the causative agent or agents, rather than changing the syndrome, throw out the supposed causative agents and find one that explained the observations better. As we know, this has not happened." (SSO p.24)

Culshaw decried the bogus logic behind the universal celebration of protease inhibitors, noting that " . . . the proportion of AIDS cases that resulted in death experienced a large drop in 1993-1994, which orthodoxy and the mass media were more than happy to portray as decreased mortality thanks to protease inhibitors. However, protease inhibitors were not even generally available to AIDS patients until 1996, over two years after the decline in the death rate began." (SSO p.27) She challenged the notion that they had been proved to extend life and argued that one only had to look at the packet inserts to see that they could "cause debilitating side effects, some of which are indistinguishable from the symptoms of AIDS itself." (SSO p.27)

She was horrified by the insane logic of HIV drug manufacturers who would insist "that since someone who was healthy when they started therapy happened to stay healthy for some time on the drugs, that is some sort of credit to the medications." (SSO p.28) She warned that "there is no evidence to say that they would not have remained healthy even if they never took any medication at all." (SSO p.28) She noted that the HIV establishment had basically gamed the system by never using placebo-controls so that it could not be determined if nothing was actually better than the AIDS drugs. "Do no harm" was a quaint joke from the distant past. As far as the reports of the supposedly positive effects upon very sick people who took the drugs, she pointed out, as others had, that reverse transcriptase inhibitors are non-specific cell-killers an in addition to harming healthy cells, could be attacking "those cells that are dividing fastest," (SSO p.28) such as the opportunistic bacteria and fungi that were the cause of acute illnesses in AIDS patients. In other words, their reputation was based on the mistaken impression that it was their effect on HIV rather than the other infections involved in the syndrome. She noted that protease inhibitors had been shown to control two of the more important infections associated with AIDS: candida and pneumocystis. (SSO p.28)

Culshaw came down hard on the absurd Orwellian invention of the term "Immune Recon stitution Syndrome" which was used to explain away the development of opportunistic infections that occurred when people were taking the miraculous protease inhibitors. The convenient ad hoc explanation was that the immune system of AIDS patients was getting "confused" as it was getting stronger. She slapped that one down, writing that "In reality, it seems to be just another attempt to explain away the fact that clearly the medications are nor working as they were intended. . . ." (SSO p.29) She zeroed in on one of the disturbing consequences of all this, one that supports our notion that the whole era should be called Holocaust II: "Consider also that the leading cause of death among medicated HIV-positives is no longer even an AIDS-defining disease at all, but liver failure, a well-documented effect of protease inhibitors." (SSO p.30)

Throughout Holocaust II, where there was AIDS there was also state coercion (the social and political face of totalitarian science) sponsored by the inexorable public health logic of the HIV/AIDS establishment. Culshaw noted, "Infants born to HIV-positive mothers are in many states forced to undergo anti-retroviral therapy and since only a few drugs have been approved for children, the drugs administered are the most toxic, AZT and nevirapine being foremost. Oftentimes this drug regimen begins before the baby is born, in certain cases against the wishes of the mother, and continues throughout childhood." (SSO p.30) And the tragedy was cruelly compounded by the fact that half of HIV-positive babies revert to negative in any case. Unforgivable iatrogenic scars from this age of medical atrocities were everywhere. (Hopefully, historians will do a good job one day of documenting them all for posterity.)

In terms of the real underlying pandemic of HHV-6, it is interesting that Culshaw zeroed in on the politically motivated nature of concocting a definition of AIDS as a disease characterized mainly by the decline in CD4+ cells: "But what was known from the beginning of AIDS—though bizarrely, not investigated to nearly the extent that CD4+ cells have been investigated—was that AIDS patients suffered disruptions in many subsets of their blood cells. [emphasis mine]. Virtually all of these patients had elevated levels of many different types of antibodies, indicating that something had gone wrong with the "antibody-arm of the immune system." (SSO p.33) (God forbid that they had looked at what was going on in the "antibody arm of the immune system" of the CFS patients and the rest of the general population.)

In her book, as she had done in her previous essay, she emphasized that the HIV tests themselves were an unreliable technical mess and was horrified at how diagnostics that were "some of the worst tests ever manufactured in terms of standardization, specificity, and reproducibility" (SSO p.35) were being used "as a weapon of discrimination ever since testing began." (SSO p.35) Everything about the way viral proteins were identified as belonging to HIV she found questionable. She described one of the common tests (the ELISA): " . . . the proteins are present in a mixture and the serum reacts with the proteins in such a way as to cause a color change. The color change is not discrete—meaning that everyone has varying degrees of reaction." (SSO p.39) It gets totally Alice-in-Wonderlandish as she notes that "there are varying degrees of the color change, and a cutoff value has been established, above which the sample is considered reactive or 'positive' and below which it is considered 'negative.' Clearly, this language is absurd, since positive and negative are polarities and not positions on a sliding scale." (SSO p.39) Such was the crazy way medical tests were conducted in the reign of abnormal science that was Holocaust II.

Culshaw also noted that everyone could test positive for HIV, depending on how the serum was diluted when the tests were run. She was inadvertently saying more about the catastrophic effects of HHV-6 on the body when she pointed out that the tests were actually detecting the previously mentioned condition of hypergammaglobinemia, or "having too many antibodies to too many things." (SSO p.44) Again it must be pointed out that, unknown to her and her colleagues in AIDS dissent, the biomedical face of the complex HHV-6 catastrophe was simultaneously revealing itself in the widespread chronic fatigue syndrome epidemic in the form of people "having too many antibodies to too many things."

The other thing which she pointed out which connected with the oft-detected evidence of retroviral activity in CFS was the possibility that the

HIV test was simply detecting endogenous retroviral activity, hence just an artifact (or epiphenomenon) of the biological chaos that was going on in the bodies of AIDS patients. The retroviral activity could be "Simply a marker for cell decay and/or division." (SSO p.44) (And, in the case of HHV-6's devastation, we know there was and is a lot of that going on.) And, again, the fact that the HIV tests had never been "validated against the gold standard of HIV isolation" (SSO p.45) decimated their credibility. Or should have

Culshaw could see that the slovenly and shady science of HIV had led America and the rest of the world into an ethical quagmire: "Since the diagnosis HIV-positive carries with it such a stigma and the potential for outrageous denial of human rights, it is only humane that doctors, AIDS researchers, and test manufacturers would want to make absolutely certain that the tests they are promoting are completely verifiable in the best possible way. This is not happening." (SSO p.45) Like some of the other HIV critics, she pointed out that the retrovirus had never been unquestionably isolated in an irrefutable way in the first place—and still hadn't been, potentially making AIDS one of the biggest scientific mistakes and scandals in history. She reinforced the point, writing, "You might think that with hundreds of billions of dollars spent so far on HIV, there would have been by now a scientific attempt to demonstrate HIV isolation by publication of proper electron micrographs. The fact that there has not indicates quite strongly that no one has been able to do it." (SSO p.46)

In addition to the HIV test not working reliably, she also questioned the viral load test, which is used "to estimate the health status of those already diagnosed HIV-positive" because "there is good reason to believe it does not work at all." (SSO p.46) She pointed to a paper that indicated "fully one-half of . . . patients with detectable viral loads had no evidence of virus by culture." (SSO p.47) It was as if the Three Stooges were in charge of every aspect of HIV testing. Culshaw was uniquely sensitive to the ugly political nature of all this and perceptively saw how the HIV tests "are used essentially as weapons of terror." (SSO p.48) She writes, "This medical terrorism reached new heights in June, 2006 with the CDC's new HIV testing guidelines, which recommended that everyone between the ages of thirteen and sixty-five be tested for antibodies to HIV." (SSO p.48)

Culshaw was outraged that the faulty test for a virus not proven to cause AIDS could force perfectly healthy people "into undergoing a regimen that will inevitably cause long-term toxic effects (and even death), a more sinister complication is the violation in human rights that occurs following a positive HIV test. Every state in the U.S. and every province in

Canada maintain a list of 'HIV carriers' in that region."(SSO p.49) That was just one more aspect of Holocaust II that made it seem very much like Holocaust I.

Culshaw could see the heavy political hands that were keeping the hellish paradigm and draconian public health agenda in place. When they were confronted by criticism grounded in logic and reason, "The AIDS orthodoxy's only counters to the points made and the questions raised consist of ad hominem attacks including use of the term 'denialist' as well as stating that dissenting views have 'long since been discredited' without any reference to exactly where these views have been discredited. Unfortunately, words are powerful and personal attacks are very effective at silencing people." (SSO p.60) She felt that it was a campaign of "fear, discrimination, and terror that has been waged aggressively by a powerful group of people whose sole motivation was and is behavior control." (SSO p.60) Of course, those would be the lucky ones. The dead ones would have no behavioral issues.

More than any other AIDS critic, she came the closest to seeing the heterosexist and racist underpinnings of the whole creepy game: "To understand the sociological motivations behind the HIV/AIDS paradigm, one must understand the racism and homophobia that has persisted in society for centuries. It is only very recently in the timeline of history that gays and blacks have been accorded equal rights under the law. . . ." (SSO p.61) Her thinking supported my contention that what the law can give gays and blacks with one hand, epidemiology in the form of homodemiology and Afrodemiology can take away with the other.

Culshaw came breathtakingly close to seeing both the forest and the trees insofar as she called it a rush to judgment at the beginning of the epidemic when the first cases of AIDS were assumed to be sexually transmitted even though the original gay men with it had no contact with each other. She was onto the heterosexist or homodemiological lenses through which the original ground zero data was being observed by the VD- and gay-obsessed pioneers of the HIV/AIDS paradigm. And she recognized that the assumption of sexual transmission was not easily dialed back or reconsidered. In terms of the HHV-6 catastrophe it is of interest that she recognized that "Despite the fact the other viruses (cytomegalovirus and herpes virus, to give two examples) were far more prevalent in AIDS patients than HIV ever was, the HIV train started rolling and hasn't lost momentum since. Would this have happened if the first AIDS patients had been heterosexuals in the prime of their lives?" (SSO p.62)

One of the most admirable things about Rebecca Culshaw is the fact that she was not afraid to use the fierce polemical language of moral indignation when confronting the reign of pseudoscientific evil: "Many of the biggest crimes committed by the AIDS orthodoxy are psychosocial and not medical at all." (SSO p.62) What the charlatans of AIDS in their white coats were doing to humanity was not something she—unlike most of her fellow scientists and intellectuals—could look away from: "The discrimination leveled against those given the HIV-positive diagnosis has reached a level not seen since leprosy was common . . . HIV-positives are the modern equivalent of lepers (and in Cuba, where they are quarantined, are even treated as such) . . ." (SSO p.63) The enforcers of the paradigm were "vultures who will stop at nothing to prop up their paradigm." (SSO p.65) While Culshaw, unfortunately, didn't see the full nature of Holocaust II as clearly as she might have, she came closer than many, and what she did see she translated into an historically important outcry: "The HIV theory has never been about science but rather about behavioral modification primarily, and to a lesser extent, about money, power and prestige. Language surrounding HIV and AIDS is infected with a sort of pious moralism that is completely inappropriate in science. . . ."(SSO p.69) Maybe inappropriate for normal science, but it is the theme song constantly playing in the background of the abnormal science of Holocaust II.

Culshaw could see that, tragically, there was no turning back, because "First of all, there are tremendous financial and social interests involved. Billions of dollars in research funding, stock options, and activist budgets are predicated on the assumptions that HIV causes AIDS. Entire industries of pharmaceutical drugs, diagnostic testing and activist causes would have no reason to exist." (SSO p.70) If that doesn't sound like an empire of evil worthy of being called Holocaust II, I don't know what does.

Few saw the costs and consequences of the HIV theory being wrong and articulated them as dramatically as Culshaw. It wasn't a small inconsequential scientific matter, a minor wrong turn that could be easily forgiven or forgotten: ". . . the scientific and medical communities have a great deal of face to lose. It is not much of an exaggeration to state that when the HIV/AIDS hypothesis is finally recognized as wrong, the entire institution of science will lose the public's trust, and science itself will experience fundamental, profound and long-lasting changes. The 'scientific community' has risked its credibility by standing by the HIV theory so long. This is why doubting the HIV hypothesis is now tantamount to doubting science itself, and this is why dissidents face excommunication." (SSO p.70) And she wasn't even aware that the fiasco included among its consequences, chronic fatigue syndrome, autism and many other "mysterious" epidemics that are being caused by HHV-6.

Culshaw is fairly unique among the Duesbergians and other HIV critics, dissidents, resistance intellectuals, whatever one wants to call them. Not only was she patently not heterosexist, not only did she not spin her own alternative "Got-AIDS-Yet, GRID-think" alternative lifestyle theory of AIDS, but she actually went in the opposite direction and argued that heterosexism, side-by-side with racism, was the driving force for the biomedical dystopia that was created by the pseudoscientific HIV/AIDS paradigm. And, in a near miss, Rebecca Culshaw almost got it right when she wrote that "powerful psychological forces are at work. It is simply easier for most people to project our neglect of disenfranchised groups— gay men, drug users, blacks, the poor and so on—onto a virus and accept those "infected" as sacrificial victims, than to recognize that there is no bug. For society, the latter would require acceptance of those disenfranchised groups as equal participants in mainstream society and culture." (SSO p.70) She would have won the "understanding Holocaust II lottery" if only she had written, "It is simply easier for most people to project our neglect of disenfranchised groups—gay men, drugs users, blacks, the poor and so on (and ignore the threat to our own health)—onto the wrong, politically and fraudulently framed virus and accept those labeled and scapegoated as "AIDS infected" and as sacrificial victims, than to recognize that we are all at risk for the real cause of this epidemic." But it was not to be. She certainly got the business about the bigoted politics right, but there was a virus, a very serious and deadly virus, but not a retrovirus. It was a DNA virus, one that was, even as she wrote her wonderful book, having its pathological way with both franchised and disenfranchised groups all over the world.

If one were to ask all the Duesbergians—including Culshaw—if the egregious errors of the AIDS medical establishment had put the heterosexual general population in more danger of becoming immune-compromised, they all would probably have said a resounding "No!" The fact that they would have been absolutely wrong (considering the HHV-6 spectrum catastrophe in the general population that was masked by the HIV "mistake") shows that their critical brilliance and their unique ethical bravery went only so far in the search for the ultimate truth about the epidemic. They failed to stop the forces of heterosexism and racism that crystallized into Holocaust II, but without all of them, our very dark time would be even darker.